Understanding Social Anxiety

Volume 153, Sage Library of Social Research

RECENT VOLUMES IN SAGE LIBRARY OF SOCIAL RESEARCH

Understanding Social Anxiety

Social, Personality, and Clinical Perspectives

Mark R. Leary

VOLUME 153
SAGE LIBRARY OF
SOCIAL RESEARCH

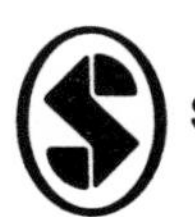

SAGE PUBLICATIONS Beverly Hills / London / New Delhi

For information address:

SAGE Publications, Inc.
275 South Beverly Drive
Beverly Hills, California 90212

SAGE Publications India Pvt. Ltd.
C-236 Defence Colony
New Delhi 110 024, India

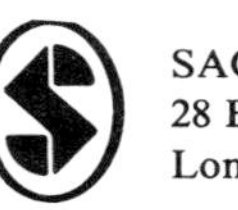

SAGE Publications Ltd
28 Banner Street
London EC1Y 8QE, England

Printed in the United States of America

Library of Congress Cataloging in Publication Data

Leary, Mark R.
Understanding social anxiety.

(Sage library of social research ; v. 153)
Bibliography: p.
Includes indexes.
1. Anxiety—Social aspects. 2. Self. 3. Social role. 4. Personality. I. Title. II. Series.
HM291.L358 1983 302'.15 83-17722
ISBN 0-8039-2165-9
ISBN 0-8039-2166-7 (pbk.)

FIRST PRINTING

CONTENTS

PREFACE

Students often have great difficulty identifying topics on which to do original research, whether for class projects, independent studies, theses, or dissertations. When talking to students who are in the throes of finding research ideas, I sometimes have a hard time convincing them that there is not just one right way to find a topic and that social scientists often stumble upon their research interests in chance and seemingly "nonscientific" ways. My interest in the topic of social anxiety is a case in point.

While eating breakfast one morning in 1979, I happened to turn to ABC's *Good Morning America* television program just in time to see host David Hartman interviewing Stanford psychologist Philip Zimbardo. As many readers undoubtedly know, Zimbardo has conducted extensive research on the topic of shyness and has written a best-selling paperback about shyness. I recall few details of the interview itself, but I remember being struck by the fact that although shyness is a very common and problematic experience for many people, I had never come across a single research article on the topic. (There were a few papers at the time, but I did not know of them.) It seemed to me that psychologists had virtually neglected an important area for basic research and applied practice.

At the time, I was working with Barry Schlenker at the University of Florida in the area of self-presentation, and I quickly became very intrigued by shyness because of its apparent relationship with people's concerns about how they are being perceived and evaluated by others. At its core, shyness seemed to arise from certain kinds of self-presentational concerns. Unfortunately, my initial literature searches were unproductive to say the least. Aside from the work of Zimbardo and his students, I found only a few papers under the heading of "shyness," leading me to conclude that the area had indeed been neglected.

Only months later did I realize that researchers were using several different terms to refer to feelings of apprehension and nervousness in social situations. Having recognized this, it was easy to locate dozens of studies dealing with constructs such as dating anxiety, speech anxiety, stagefright, communication apprehension, audience anxiety, embarrassment, heterosocial anxiety, interpersonal anxiety, and, of course, *social anxiety.* Not surprisingly, articles on these topics were scattered throughout the journals of a number of areas of behavioral science, ranging from psychology to speech communication.

The present volume was born of the clear need for an integrated review of these diverse bodies of research. The keyword here is *integrated.* It is encouraging to me that there is a trend toward integrating areas of behavioral science that have often treated one another as strangers, and particularly between so-called basic and applied areas. Witness volumes such as *Integrations of Clinical and Social Psychology* (Weary & Mirels, 1982) and the newly formed *Journal of Social and Clinical Psychology.* There are many topics—and I believe social anxiety is one—in which full understanding cannot be attained without interconnecting theory, research, and practice across a number of diverse areas. Thus, this book is intended to integrate and review the literatures on social anxiety from social, personality, and clinical perspectives. It is my hope that the integrated product is equally palatable to researchers and practitioners in all relevant areas.

In writing this book I kept four kinds of readers in mind. First, researchers in various areas of psychology and speech communication who have an interest in social anxiety and related constructs will find the book useful. Although it is not intended as an exhaustive, encyclopedic treatment of social anxiety, I have covered some of the central issues and problems in sufficient detail to please researchers who are already quite familiar with the existing literature. Second, as a high proportion of people who seek professional help for personal difficulties are troubled by feelings of social anxiety, many practitioners in psychology and speech communication should find the book relevant to their work. Not only is social anxiety placed within a theoretical framework for maximal understanding, but implications for the assessment and treatment of problematic social anxiousness are discussed throughout the book. In the same vein, professional courses in counseling and clinical psychology should find the book relevant.

Understanding Social Anxiety might be used as a supplemental text for a variety of courses in social, personality, clinical, and counseling psychology. Not only does it provide the student with an overview of an important and inherently interesting psychological phenomenon, it also demonstrates the interconnections among what students often perceive as unrelated subareas of behavioral science. It shows the applicability of "basic" theory and research to clinical practice and the reciprocal impact of "applied" work on basic understanding. The book is particularly appropriate for the growing number of courses dealing specifically with integrations of clinical-counseling and social-personality psychology.

Finally, although the book is intended as a scholarly treatment of the topic, the reader with a personal rather than professional interest in social anxiety should find it inherently interesting. It has been my experience that nearly everyone is intrigued by a scientific examination of the prevalent, mundane experience of social anxiety.

Many people share partial responsibility for this book. Foremost is Barry Schlenker who has made an indelible mark upon both my professional and personal growth. Much of my work on social anxiety has been in collaboration with Barry and he deserves full credit for many of the ideas in this book. I would also like to thank the people at Sage Publications for their support and guidance throughout the writing and editing process and two excellent reviewers for their insights and suggestions. Knowing that it is *de rigueur* to acknowledge the support of one's spouse during the writing of a book, I want to be sure that the full extent of Wendy's contribution is recognized. Beyond her patience and unflagging support, her help as a live-in reviewer, critic, and editor were of immeasurable value. I might have never gotten the whole thing off the ground had it not been for the hospitality of Bill and Anne Cutlip who, on more than one occasion, allowed me to hide-out and work at their home where I could be free of distractions. Initial work on the book was facilitated by a Summer Professional Development Grant from Denison University. Many thanks to my former colleagues and students at Denison.

—Mark R. Leary

1

THE CONSTRUCT OF SOCIAL ANXIETY

Stop for a moment and visualize, as vividly as you can, each of the following scenarios:

You are about to deliver a speech to an audience of several hundred. As you peek out at the packed auditorium from backstage, you mentally kick yourself for not having prepared and rehearsed your talk as adequately as you had planned. You look at your watch and see that it's three minutes until you walk out on that big, empty stage (hoping to appear relaxed, coordinated, and poised in the process) and adjust the microphone. Microphone?! You can imagine your voice booming back at you from the far corners of the hall, interrupting your thoughts and paralyzing your speech. You lick your lips and look at your watch again: one minute to go.

You are at a party where you know only a few of the other guests. Unfortunately, they are currently engaged in a conversation in another room. So you stand there, trying not to look as out of place as you feel. You sip your drink and smile (rather foolishly you think) at other guests as they pass. A conversation starts up near you, so you saunter over and attempt to join in, but your interjections are met only with nods and polite smiles. It is clear that the others are not interested in what you have to say and some even appear to resent your intrusion into what appears, on second thought, to have been an intimate conversation. So, you stand there (looking very foolish, you think again) and try to appear interested and relaxed, although you're not.

If you have never found yourself in social situations like these in which you felt anxious, uncertain, self-conscious, and awkward, you are a highly unusual person. All available evidence indicates that nearly everyone experiences anxiety and apprehension in social situations from time to time. Over 90% of the American respondents surveyed by Zimbardo (1977; Zimbardo, Pilkonis, & Norwood, 1974) indicated that they felt shy at least occasionally, and over 50% reported that shyness sometimes constituted a significant problem for them. Similarly, studies have found that between 11% and 37% of college students (depending upon the particular study) express some degree of apprehension about interacting with or dating members of the other sex (e.g., Borkovec, Stone, O'Brien, & Kaloupek, 1974; Glass, Gottman, & Schmurak, 1976; Arkowitz, Hinton, Perl, & Himadi, 1978). In fact, Martinson and Zerface (1970) reported that respondents in their college sample were more interested in obtaining help for their concerns about dealing with the other sex than they were in seeking assistance for academic and precareer problems. A great variety of mundane events cause feelings of social anxiety in a high proportion of the population, including interactions with strangers, job interviews, being the center of attention, and talking to authority figures. Social anxiety aroused by the prospect of public speaking is perhaps the most prevalent. The fear of speaking before large groups is the most commonly reported fear among both college students and the general public (Bruskin Associates, 1973; Bryant & Trower, 1974; Geer, 1965). McCroskey (1970, 1977) estimates that at least 20% of American college students may be characterized as having a high degree of communication apprehension, and it is likely that fear of public speaking may be even more common in the population at large. In short, socially based anxiety is very common.

Given the prevalence of social anxiety and the degree to which many people consider such feelings to be personally problematic, one might guess that behavioral scientists would have devoted considerable research attention to the topic. On the contrary, with a few notable exceptions (e.g., Clevinger, 1959; Dixon, de Monchaux, & Sandler, 1957; Gilkinson, 1942, 1943; Paul, 1966; Watson & Friend, 1969), little research was conducted in the area until the early 1970s. However, since then a large body of research has emerged although it has not always been published under the heading of "social anxiety." Researchers from the various specialty areas of psychology and speech communication seem to have a penchant for using different terms to refer to the experience of apprehension and anxiety in social settings. As a result, the literature is littered with terms such as dating anxiety, speech anxiety, shyness, interpersonal anxiety, heterosexual-social anxiety, stagefright, communication apprehension, embarrassment, and audience anxiety, to name the most common. Lest the reader be misled, let me note that these terms are not, strictly speaking, synonymous with one another. Nevertheless, they all seem to be associated with the more general construct of social anxiety, as we shall see throughout this book.

Because research on social anxiety has appeared under these various guises and in the journals of a number of diverse specialty areas (chiefly social, personality, counseling, and clinical psychology, and speech communication), there have been relatively few attempts to integrate these isolated pockets of research (see, however, Buss, 1980; Leary & Schlenker, 1981; Schlenker & Leary, 1982). In many cases, researchers in each of these areas have carried on their own lines of work, seemingly oblivious to intimately related research from other areas. (I include myself among the offenders.) In recognition of this state of affairs, one of my goals in writing this volume is to review and integrate the growing literatures on social anxiety.

Social Anxiety: A Definition

One reason for the fragmentation of social anxiety research is that few writers have attempted to provide explicit definitions of the constructs under study. Without a clear conceptualization of an umbrella construct under which to gather the various "forms" of social anxiety (such as shyness, dating anxiety, stagefright, and so on), researchers have often failed to recognize the connections between their research and that of others and between the focus of their work and the broader construct of social anxiety. Thus, let me first propose a working definition of social anxiety that both identifies the nature of the experience and that subsumes each of the closely related constructs listed above.

As we will use it here, social anxiety is defined as "anxiety resulting from the prospect or presence of interpersonal evaluation in real or imagined social settings" (Schlenker & Leary, 1982, p. 642). For clarity, it is necessary to discuss briefly the components of this definition and to contrast it with others' definitions of social anxiety and related constructs.

ANXIETY

As tautological as it may sound, it is important to note that I define social anxiety as a state of *anxiety*. Interestingly, other writers have not always defined social anxiety precisely in this manner. In particular, many definitions include patterns of inhibited or avoidant behavior as characteristics of the phenomenon. To quote only one example, Watson and Friend (1969) defined social-evaluative anxiety as the "experience of distress, discomfort, fear, anxiety, etc. in social situations; as the deliberate avoidance of social situations; and... as a fear of receiving negative evaluations from others" (p. 448; see also Buss, 1980; Clark & Arkowitz, 1975). Such definitions are problematic because, as shall be explored in Chapter 6, there is not a necessary relationship between subjective feelings of social anxiety and overt patterns of avoidant or inhibited behavior. While it is true that people who feel nervous in social settings show a tendency to become reticent, inhibited, and avoidant, people may feel quite anxious without displaying any of these behaviors (Leary, 1982; McCroskey, 1977). Thus, it makes little sense to define anxiety in behavioral terms.

In addition to creating conceptual confusion, including behavioral criteria in definitions of social anxiety raises important questions about measurement (Leary, 1983a, 1983c). If we wish to measure an individual's level of social anxiety, should we measure affect, behavior, or both? Can we use behavioral measures of a subjective state? These are more than hypothetical queries.

As will be seen below, many self-report measures of dispositional social anxiousness confound the measurement of social anxiety with the measurement of behavioral responses that sometimes accompany the experience (Leary, 1982, 1983a; McCroskey, 1977). Even more problematic are studies that use *purely* behavioral measures of social anxiety. In addition to obfuscating the interpretation of the data obtained from such measures, the failure to distinguish between anxiety and behavior makes it impossible to explore questions regarding the relationship *between* subjectively experienced social anxiety and interpersonal behavior. It seems to me most sensible to define and measure social anxiety independently of specific overt behaviors and then empirically examine the relationship between the two (see Chapter 6).

Anxiety itself has been a problematic construct in psychology for many years (Speilberger, 1966). However, I think that most would agree that anxiety may be defined, roughly, as a cognitive-affective syndrome that is characterized by physiological arousal (indicative of sympathetic nervous system arousal) and apprehension or dread regarding an impending, potentially negative outcome that the person believes he or she is unable to avert (cf. Dixon et al., 1957; Paul & Bernstein, 1973; Schlenker & Leary, 1982). Some writers have attempted to distinguish between the concepts of anxiety and fear (see Epstein, 1967), but I would side with those who advocate abolishing what appears to be a somewhat artificial distinction. There does not seem to be any compelling theoretical reason to maintain the anxiety-fear distinction (Izard & Tomkins, 1966; Lesse, 1970), at least not when speaking of *social* concerns. We will use the term "anxiety" rather than "fear" throughout this book since virtually all writers in the area have done so.

THE NATURE OF SOCIAL ANXIETY

There are nearly an infinite number and variety of events and objects that cause people to become anxious. People may be afraid to fly in airplanes, apprehensive about dealing with spiders or snakes, or worried when they must walk down a deserted city street at night. They may experience anxiety when giving a speech, taking an important examination, sitting in the waiting room at the dentist's office, or starting the first day of a new job. (The reader will be able to generate his or her personal list of objects and events that are particularly threatening. More than likely, the list includes the grim reaper in one guise or another.) Given the many causes of anxiety, two questions must be addressed. Is there any justification for regarding socially based anxieties as a distinct subclass of anxiety and, if so, on what basis may social anxiety be distinguished from anxiety due to other causes?

Obviously, if I didn't think that the answer to the first question is "yes," I wouldn't have written this book; there appears to be merit in distinguishing a class of social anxieties among the plethora of anxieties people experience. Numerous studies have presented subjects with lists of anxiety-producing stimuli and asked them how anxious, fearful, or nervous they feel when they confront each stimulus. When respondents' ratings are factor analyzed, all studies have obtained solutions that include at least one category of what has been labeled "social" or "interpersonal" anxieties (Bates, 1971; Bernstein & Allen, 1969; Braun & Reynolds, 1969; Endler, Hunt, & Rosenstein, 1962; Landy & Gaupp, 1971; Lawlis, 1971; Strahan, 1974), including one study of children's fears (Miller, Barrett, Hampe, & Noble, 1972). Although each of these studies used different lists of anxiety-evoking stimuli and obtained somewhat different factor structures, all of them identified at least one factor that reflected interpersonal concerns. Thus, it appears that social settings constitute a discrete class of anxiety-producing stimuli.

Turning, then, to the second question: What is it that socially based anxieties have in common that distinguish them from other sources of anxiety? It isn't enough to suggest that social anxiety is distinguishable by virtue of the fact that it is experienced in social as opposed to other types of situations although some writers have defined it in this way. Being accosted by an angry drunk while at a party would be an example of an anxiety-provoking event that, presumably, we would not want to label as social anxiety, despite the fact that it was experienced in a social setting.

An examination of the kinds of situations that load heavily on the social anxiety factors in the studies described above provides some clues regarding the essence of social anxiety. These include: being introduced to new people, dating someone for the first time, being interviewed for a job, giving a speech, being the center of attention, entering a roomful of strangers, being tested, talking to people in positions of authority, and being ridiculed, to name some of the commonly obtained items. This list of social anxiety items is nearly identical to the list of shyness-producing situations obtained in Zimbardo's (1977) extensive survey research.

What these kinds of situations seem to have in common is that they all involve the prospect or presence of *interpersonal evaluation,* a characteristic not shared by other sources of anxiety (Schlenker & Leary, 1982). In other instances of anxiety—facing the prospect of losing one's job, being followed by a person who appears to be a mugger, having family problems, and so on—the anxiety is not precipitated by concerns about the evaluation of oneself by others. In the case of social anxiety, such concerns predominate.

But why should the prospect or presence of interpersonal evaluation cause people to feel anxious? As I will explain in greater detail in Chapter 3, during the course of social encounters people continually form impressions of and evaluate one another. In some instances, the evaluation is explicit (as when one is being interviewed for a job or is giving a political campaign speech). More often, the evaluations are implicit and not overtly acknowledged by any of the parties involved. These impressions and accompanying evaluations play a large role in determining how the participants in social encounters respond to one another (Goffman, 1959; Schlenker, 1980; Snyder, Tanke, & Berscheid, 1977). Positive evaluations of an individual are likely to result in positive social outcomes, whereas the formation of negative evaluations typically results in less positive if not clearly negative responses from others. Since the evaluations of others determine in large part how people are treated by other people, most individuals are generally motivated to be evaluated as positively as possible by those with whom they deal. According to the definition of social anxiety presented above, it is this concern with interpersonal evaluation that causes people to feel socially anxious under certain circumstances (Leary, 1980, 1982; Leary & Schlenker, 1981; Schlenker & Leary, 1982; Zimbardo, 1977).

As we will see throughout the book, most research evidence strongly supports the conceptualization of social anxiety as being precipitated by concerns with the interpersonal evaluation of oneself by others. For example, in a study of 35 individuals who sought professional help for very problematic social anxiousness, Nichols (1974) found that the central characteristic of these individuals was hypersensitivity to and fearfulness of disapproval and criticism from others. Similarly, people who are highly concerned about how they are evaluated by others are much more likely to experience social anxiety than people who are less apprehensive about others' evaluations (Leary, 1983a; Watson & Friend, 1969). In addition, episodes of social anxiety are generally accompanied by the expectation that one will make an unfavorable impression and be evaluated negatively by other interactants, whether or not this is actually the case (e.g., Glass et al., 1976; Leary, 1980; Rehm & Marston, 1968).

Many existing definitions of social anxiety indicate that social anxiety occurs "in the presence of others" or "while interacting with others." On the contrary, social anxiety may occur even when other people are *not* present. (Just ask any adolescent who has ever had the jitters while getting ready for a "big date" or the speaker who feels nervous while rehearsing his or her speech alone.) In many cases, extreme anxiety may result from simply imagining a social scenerio that may not ever come to pass. People may feel nervous just from thinking about an upcoming date, a job interview, an impending speech, tomorrow night's cocktail party with the boss, and so on. For this reason, the definition of social anxiety presented above notes that social anxiety may result from the *prospect or presence* of interpersonal evaluation in *real or imagined* social settings (cf. McCroskey's 1977 definition of communication apprehension).

The latest edition of the *Diagnostic and Statistical Manual of Mental Disorders* (*DSM*-III) includes a psychiatric construct that is conceptually quite similar to the present definition of social anxiety. According to the *DSM*-III (1980, p. 227), *social phobia* is

> a persistent, irrational fear of, and compelling desire to avoid, situations in which the individual may be exposed to the scrutiny of others. There is also fear that the individual will behave in a manner that will be humiliating or embarrassing. Marked anticipatory anxiety occurs if the individual is confronted with the necessity of entering such a situation, and he or she therefore attempts to avoid it.

Defined in this manner, social phobia may be regarded as chronic and severe social anxiousness. Four points should be noted about the definition of social phobia. First, consistent with the present approach, the definition locates the source of the experience in the individual's concerns with others' "scrutiny." Second, it acknowledges that the experience may be anticipatory in nature, sometimes occurring in the absence of other people. Third, this definition departs from our definition of social anxiety in that it includes both affective and behavioral (avoidance) responses as defining characteristics of social phobia. We have already discussed problems associated with defining a subjective phenomenon in terms of behavior. An individual who often became terrified in social encounters but who forced him- or herself to participate in them would not be classified as socially phobic. Finally, the *DSM*'s definition refers to social phobia as an "irrational" fear; reactions are typically labeled "phobic" when the degree of anxiety experienced is out of proportion to the objective degree of threat involved. Unfortunately, the *DSM* provides no criteria for judging whether or not the individual's fear of others' scrutiny is rational or irrational. For now, let us simply note that there is nothing inherently irrational about being concerned about others' scrutiny and evaluations, and that the term social phobia should probably be reserved for only the most extreme cases of social anxiety. In line with this recommendation, Nichols (1974) disputes the idea that most instances of social anxiety should be considered phobic.

Introversion, Sociability, and Reticence

Having defined what social anxiety is, let me say a few words about what it is not. As it has been defined here, social anxiety is a subjectively experienced state. However, the construct has sometimes been confused with the behavioral constructs of introversion, sociability, and reticence. Although each of these constructs is, in some way, related to social anxiety, it is important to distinguish between them.

INTROVERSION

Introversion refers to a preference for solitary, rather than gregarious activities. Introverts typically prefer to be alone, are quiet and retiring, tend to be introspective and cautious, and have primarily solitary interests. At the opposite end of the continuum, extraverts are sociable, enjoy interacting with others, often enjoy taking risks, and are outgoing (Eysenck & Eysenck, 1969; Eysenck & Rachman, 1965).

Although there is a correlation between introversion and social anxiety (e.g., Cheek & Buss, 1981; Pilkonis, 1977a; Watson & Friend, 1969), the two constructs are not isomorphic. It cannot be assumed that introverted individuals are necessarily socially anxious. Many introverts simply find it more rewarding to pursue activities that do not involve other people but are not unusually anxious when they interact with others. Henry David Thoreau, for example, preferred a solitary lifestyle for two years at Walden Pond, but does not appear to have been particularly socially anxious on those occasions when he interacted with others. As an introvert, Thoreau simply saw little value in frequent social encounters:

> Society is commonly too cheap. We meet at very short intervals, not having had time to acquire any new value for each other. We meet at three meals a day and give each other a taste of that old musty cheese that we are. We have had to agree on a certain set of rules, called etiquette and politeness, to make this frequent meeting tolerable and that we need not come to open war. . . . Cer-

tainly less frequency would suffice for all important and hearty communication [Thoreau, 1962: 206].

Although introversion-extraversion and social anxiety are conceptually distinguishable, there is evidence that they are correlated (Huntley, 1969; Pilkonis, 1977a). In some instances, introverted lifestyles may arise from a tendency to become socially anxious in interpersonal encounters. It is not surprising that people who are often anxious in social settings will prefer doing other kinds of things. Even so, introversion per se refers only to a preference for nonsocial activities and does not involve social anxiety.

SOCIABILITY

Closely related to introversion-extraversion is the concept of sociability. Sociability is defined as the preference for affiliating with others rather than being alone. Highly sociable people like to be with others, welcome the opportunity to interact, prefer working with others rather than alone, and report being particularly unhappy when they are unable to make social contacts over an extended period of time (Cheek & Buss, 1981). Unsociable people, on the other hand, do not particularly enjoy or frequently engage in social activities although, it should be noted, they do not necessarily find them aversive. Thus, sociability is one component of introversion and, like introversion, is defined independently of social anxiety. Sociability is a behavioral construct; social anxiety is an affective construct that may, of course, have behavioral concomitants.

Cheek and Buss (1981) constructed separate scales to measure sociability and shyness (which they defined, roughly, as social anxiety plus inhibited behavior). Factor analyses of the responses of over 900 respondents revealed distinct sociability and shyness factors. The correlation between shyness and sociability was $-.30$ which, although statistically significant, showed that shyness and sociability are distinct constructs (see, also, Leary, 1983a).

In the second phase of their research, Cheek and Buss (1981) classified subjects as either low or high on both the shyness and sociability measures. They then examined affective and behavioral differences among the four types of subjects identified by this classification. In brief, they found that shyness and sociability independently contributed to subjects' reactions in face-to-face encounters. Interestingly, the "shy-sociable" subjects demonstrated the strongest evidence of experiencing social anxiety when interacting with others. Such individuals have a high need to interact with others (i.e., they are highly sociable), yet they feel uncomfortable and inhibited when doing so (i.e., they are shy). These competing pressures may result in further tension, awkwardness, and inhibition. Shyness is less troublesome for "unsociable" individuals who are not as strongly motivated to be gregarious. In short, research suggests that sociability and social anxiety should be regarded as conceptually independent.

RETICENCE

As originally used in the speech communication literature, reticence referred to anxiety experienced as a result of communicating with other people (see Phillips, 1968). More recently, the term reticence has been used in a manner consistent with its dictionary definition: disposed to be silent. Thus, reticence refers to a reluctance to communicate with others (Johnson, 1973; McCroskey, 1982). According to Phillips (1980, p. 11), reticent "merely describes the behavior of people who do not communicate freely and easily." Throughout this book, I will use the latter, behavioral definition of reticence. When defined in this way, reticence is clearly distinguishable from social anxiety.

The Problematic Construct of Shyness

The construct of shyness presents researchers and practitioners with a special conceptual problem because it has been defined by various authors as (a) a form of social anxiety (Buss, 1980; Leary & Schlenker, 1981; Zimbardo, 1977); (b) a pattern of avoidant, reticent, and/or inhibited behavior (Phillips, 1980; Pilkonis, 1977a); and (c) an anxiety-behavioral syndrome, characterized by feelings of anxiety *and* inhibited or avoidant behavior (Cheek & Buss, 1981; Crozier, 1979; Jones & Russell, 1982; Morris, 1982). Throughout his book on the topic, Zimbardo (1977) purposefully refrained from defining shyness, allowing instead each research participant and reader to "adopt his or her own definition" (p. 24). Although he provides no explicit definition of the construct, Zimbardo seems to favor definition (a) above, referring at more than one point in the book to the fact that shyness is a "fear of people" (p. 32).[1]

Given the ambiguous and inconsistent use of the term, it is not clear what we should do with the construct of "shyness." At minimum, researchers should be cautioned against assuming that shyness is a unitary construct or that it is defined and used consistently in the literature (McCroskey, 1982). My own thoughts on the subject have vacilated considerably over the past few years (Leary, 1980; Leary, 1983c; Leary & Schlenker, 1981). It now seems to me that, in order to avoid confusion, the term "social anxiety" should be used when referring to the subjective experience of apprehension and nervousness we have been discussing, and specific patterns of inhibited, avoidant, or reticent behavior should be explicitly described rather than be referred to loosely as "shylike" behavior. By clearly distinguishing between subjective anxiety and overt behavior, the factors affecting anxiety versus one's behavior may be more readily identified and the relationship *between* anxiety and behavior more fully explored. The term "shy" should probably be reserved for the response *syndrome* characterized by both social anxiety and inhibited interpersonal behavior, in a manner akin to its use by Cheek and Buss (1981). Thus, a shy person is one who is anxious *and* inhibited in a social setting. Given the inconsitent uses of the term "shyness" in the literature, I will try to alert the reader to the definition used in the studies I discuss.

Are There Different "Types" of Social Anxiety?

Anyone who has ever attempted a literature search using the keywords "social anxiety" is likely to have been disappointed by the relatively small number of studies that were accessed. As I noted earlier, only a portion of the studies that deal with various manifestations of social anxiety use that specific term in their titles or text. Rather, research dealing with social anxiety appears in several alternative guises, such as communication apprehension, dating anxiety, shyness, stagefright, embarrassment, and so on. When one's literature search includes these and related terms, a large body of research will be unearthed.

Do not let me mislead you into thinking that all of these terms are synonymous. They are not. Yet, despite differences in their meanings, they have all been used to refer to anxiety experienced in social settings. In most instances, the type of encounter concerned is specifically identified by the term itself (e.g., dating anxiety, stagefright). The fact that researchers have used such a variety of terms (often without seeming to realize that they were talking about the more global construct of social anxiety) raises the question of whether there is merit in distinguishing among different types or forms of social anxiety. Put another way, do these different terms reflect meaningful distinctions among different experiences, or are they simply different terms for the same general experience, albeit the same experience in different social contexts?

At one level it appears that depending upon how they are defined, all of the terms that have been used to refer to social anxiety refer to the *same* psychological phenomenon (i.e., anxiety). The different terms only serve to obscure the fact that the constructs do not refer to subjectively different experiences. Anxiety, as far as anyone has been able to discern, is anxiety, no matter where it is experienced or what triggered it. The different constructs are distinct only inasmuch as they refer to social anxiety in different kinds of social settings.

Yet, even though these terms may be considered specific instances of the umbrella construct of social anxiety, there may be some merit in distinguishing them. Buss (1980) proposed a four-way classification of types of social anxiety. He classified all instances of social anxiety as either shyness, audience anxiety, embarrassment, or shame. He defined shyness as the "relative absence of expected behavior," and audience anxiety as "fear, tension, and disorganization in front of an audience" (pp. 184, 165). Although both embarrassment and shame occur when one has failed to behave appropriately, they differ in that embarrassment is precipitated by a violation of social norms whereas shame involves an ethical or moral infraction. According to Buss, the subjective experience of embarrassment is marked by feelings of foolishness whereas shame is characterized by feelings of self-disgust and self-abasement.

Although Buss' taxonomy provides a useful scheme for organizing the research on social anxiety, it has some conceptual problems. First, his definitions of the varieties of social anxiety are not parallel. Some are defined in terms of precipitating factors, another by the nature of the subjective affective experience, and another by the individual's behavioral responses. (For example, shyness is defined in terms of overt behaviors whereas shame is defined by the nature of the infraction and accompanying subjective reaction.) Second, the basis upon which these forms of social anxiety may be distinguished from one another is not clear. Buss does not tell us what the dimension is that underlies his classification scheme.

A second classification system has been proposed by Barry Schlenker and myself (Leary & Schlenker, 1981; Schlenker & Leary, 1982). This scheme suggests that the important distinctions among types of social anxiety are based on two independent dimensions: (a) whether the social encounter is a contingent or noncontingent one, and (b) whether or not a specific self-presentational predicament has befallen the socially anxious individual. Let us briefly examine these two dimensions.

Social settings differ in the degree to which a person's behavior is dependent or contingent upon the responses of other people in the encounter (cf. Jones & Gerard, 1967). In some social settings, a person's speech and behavior are highly contingent upon what other people are saying and doing. An example of such a contingent interaction is everyday conversation. Each person engaged in the conversation must base what he or she says, at least to a degree, upon what the others have said in order for the interaction to proceed smoothly. Likewise, an applicant in a job interview must tailor his or her responses to the questions posed by the interviewer. Interactants who do not respond contingently in such encounters will be negatively evaluated and possibly shunned (Goffman, 1967). In short, when in contingent interactions, people usually have a general idea of the kinds of things they would like to say and do during the encounter, but their behavior is based on others' responses on a moment-to-moment basis.

In *noncontingent* encounters, people's responses are not based to any great degree on others' behaviors. Instead, what they say and do is guided by a preformed plan of some kind. In Abelson's (1976) terms, their behavior is strongly "scripted." For example, a woman presenting a prepared speech would be performing noncontingent responses. Her behavior is guided primarily by the prepared text of the speech and influenced minimally, if at all, by the actions of others present. In some noncontingent encounters, the person's behavior is *cued* by others' actions, but the content of their responses is not affected by what others do. For instance, an actor in a play follows a memorized script which allows little or no flexibility in her verbal responses; the lines must be delivered as rehearsed at appropriate times. However, the actions of others on stage serve a cuing function, indicating to the actor when to deliver her lines; but, the content of her speech is not contingent upon anyone else's responses.

To be perfectly precise, encounters differ on a contingent-noncontingent *continuum,* ranging from purely contingent to purely noncontingent but with most settings containing aspects of both kinds of encounters. Nevertheless, it appears useful to make the distinction between contingent and noncontingent encounters and examine the relevance of this distinction to social anxiety. The distinction is of more than taxonomic importance. First, it provides one dimension for classifying social anxieties. Some terms, such as dating anxiety, shyness, interpersonal anxiety, and heterosocial anxiety are more applicable to contingent interactions. Stagefright, speech anxiety, and audience anxiety are generally used when the encounter is a noncontingent one. (The terms communication apprehension and embarrassment are nonspecific regarding type of encounter.)

More importantly, this distinction has implications both for the classes of factors that precipitate social anxiety and for many of the typical reactions of socially anxious people. Although these will be discussed in detail in later chapters, a word of introduction is appropriate here. Certain kinds of interpersonal difficulties are more prevalent in contingent than in noncontingent encounters, and vice versa. For instance, one common cause of social anxiety is ambiguity regarding how to respond (Buss, 1980); people often feel nervous when they do not know how to behave in a particular social encounter. Such difficulties would be expected to exacerbate social anxiety primarily in contingent types of encounters. When in contingent interactions, people are required to modify their responses on the basis of others' actions and contextual cues, raising the possibility of response uncertainty at any given moment. Social ambiguity is much less likely in a noncontingent encounter since the individual's behavior is scripted. As a result, a person who has difficulties discerning how best to respond should be particularly bothered by contingent encounters of all kinds but should find noncontingent encounters less troublesome. The differences between contingent and noncontingent encounters help explain why some people are relatively comfortable in face-to-face conversations, but experience anxiety when in a noncontingent setting, and vice versa. The structures of these two types of encounters impose very different sorts of demands upon interactants. I will return to this point later.

The second dimension that may be used to classify social anxieties cross-cuts the contingent-noncontingent dimension. It regards whether the individual's anxiety was caused by a *specific* event that casts the individual in a negative light or by an unfocused anticipation of such an event occurring. In some instances, people feel socially anxious even though nothing in particular has happened that leads them to believe they will be evaluated unfavorably by others. They are simply afraid that others will not perceive them as they desire. In other encounters, social anxiety is clearly precipitated by a particular social event—a self-presentational predicament—that has resulted in potentially negative evaluations or outcomes for the individual. The social threat is perceived as immediate and having already occurred; it is not merely anticipated. When people report feeling embarrassed, for example, they are anxious because something has happened that has made them appear foolish, incompetent, immoral, unstable, or otherwise socially undesirable (Goffman, 1955; Schlenker, 1980).

Using the two dimensions just described, all instances of social anxiety may be classified according to (a) whether the encounter is contingent or noncontingent, and (b) whether or not the anxiety results from a specific self-presentational predicament. The heuristic value of these distinctions will become apparent as we proceed.

Individual Differences in Social Anxiousness

As defined earlier, social anxiety is conceptualized as a subjective *state* of anxiety aroused by certain kinds of social psychological factors. There are, of course, great differences among individuals in the frequency and intensity with which this state is experienced. Some people experience social anxiety only rarely, whereas others become socially anxious in a large number and variety of social settings. Thus, there is some merit in regarding individual differences in the tendency to experience social anxiety as a meaningful dispositional or trait variable (see, for example, Crozier, 1979). Much research has examined the cognitive, affective, and behavioral differences among people who differ on measures of dispositional or trait social anxiety, and other studies have investigated temperamental and developmental antecedents of the disposition to experience social anxiety. We will refer to this research throughout the book and will focus specifically on individual differences in social anxiousness in Chapter 7.

For now, three points should be noted. First, writers have sometimes used the term "social anxiety" to refer to both the state of social anxiety and to the disposition to experience social anxiety, which could result in confusion for the unaware reader. Fortunately, many researchers have made their uses of the terms explicit, often by calling the individual difference variable "dispositional social anxiety" or "trait social anxiety." Elsewhere, I have suggested that "social *anxiousness*" is an appropriate label for this variable (Leary, 1983a). Throughout this book, I will attempt to make my uses of the terms explicit.

Second, the literatures on social anxiety (the state) and social anxiousness (the trait) mesh nicely in that the cognitive, affective, and behavioral concomitants of social anxiety are virtually identical to the cognitive, affective, and behavioral differences observed between people identified as dispositionally high versus low in social anxiousness. Put simply, the factors associated with state social anxiety closely parallel those correlated with trait social anxiousness. Thus, in examining the experience of social anxiety, the two literatures complement one another and will be discussed together as we proceed.

Third, the reader is cautioned that the various self-report scales that have been constructed to measure individual differences in social anxiousness differ considerably from one another and often from the conceptualization of social anxiety I am proposing. As discussed earlier, one major problem is that several commonly used scales confound the measurement of social anxiousness with the measurement of specific patterns of reticent, avoidant, and/or awkward behavior, thus obscuring the meaning of their scores (Leary, 1983a). The Appendix contains very brief descriptions of seven of the most commonly used measures of social anxiousness and related constructs, including the Social Avoidance and Distress Scale (Watson & Friend, 1969), the Self-Consciousness Scale (Fenigstein, Scheier, & Buss, 1975), the Shyness Scale (Cheek & Buss, 1981), the Stanford Shyness Survey (Zimbardo, 1977), the Personal Report of Confidence as a Speaker (Paul, 1966), the Social Anxiousness Scale (Leary, 1983a), and the Personal Report of Communication Apprehension (McCroskey, 1970, 1975, 1977, 1982). These descriptions include brief reports of reliability and validity data and comments regarding the appropriateness of the scales as measures of dispositional social anxiousness. Readers who use any of these scales in their work are encouraged to examine these critiques, as is anyone who is totally unfamiliar with these measures. I will be referring to them on several occasions throughout the book.

Overview of the Book

In this chapter, I have attempted to introduce the basic concepts, issues, and distinctions that are central to understanding social anxiety. We may now turn our attention to more substantive matters. In the next chapter, I will examine and evaluate the three major theoretical approaches that have been applied to the analysis and treatment of social anxiety. As we will see, each approach accounts for many known antecedents of the experience, but none is sufficient to explain all causes. Chapter 3 introduces the reader to a social psychological theory of social anxiety that attempts to integrate earlier approaches by identifying two conditions that, together, are necessary and sufficient antecedents of all instances of social anxiety. This theory provides an excellent framework within which to examine and understand the known situational and dispositional antecedents of social anxiety. Chapters 4 and 5 examine the propositions of the theory in greater detail and review much of the existing literature in light of it.

As I mentioned earlier, when people feel socially anxious they tend to behave in certain ways. The relationship between the affective experience of social anxiety and interpersonal behavior is dealt with in Chapter 6. Chapter 7 delves more deeply into individual differences in social anxiousness, focusing on temperamental and developmental antecedents. Finally, Chapter 8 applies our understanding of social anxiety to recommendations for assessment, counseling, and research.

Note

1. The problems inherent in allowing research participants to use their own definitions of a construct, such as shyness, when answering questions are obvious. When this approach is taken, it is difficult if not impossible to know whether respondents are talking about their subjective social anxiety, behavioral inhibition and avoidance, or both. It is likely that Zimbardo's (1977) respondents interpreted some of his questions in a variety of ways.

2

THEORETICAL PERSPECTIVES

Current thinking regarding the antecedents and treatment of social anxiety may be classified, roughly, as reflecting one of three general theoretical perspectives: the conditioned anxiety, social skills deficit, or cognitive approaches. An examination of the literatures surrounding these orientations may lead one to conclude that they are competing, mutually exclusive psychological models. Many studies have pitted these approaches and their respective theory-based treatments against one another, presumably in search of *the* best theory and treatment for social anxiety. This does not appear to be a very productive strategy, however; after dozens of such studies, no one approach has emerged a clear victor.

This suggests to me that, like most psychological phenomena, social anxiety is multiply determined and that none of these approaches is able to account for all instances in which people experience social anxiety. Similarly, each treatment strategy based upon these approaches may be appropriate for some cases of problematic social anxiousness, but not for others. Thus, it does not seem judicious to regard the three approaches as mutually exclusive (Arkowitz et al., 1978; Curran, 1977). Instead, we should recognize that each perspective provides one view of the causes and treatment of social anxiety.

Classical Conditioning

Most psychologists maintain that human beings have few, if any, inborn fears or anxieties. It is true that young babies show a "startle response" to certain stimuli such as loud noises and loss of physical support (i.e., falling), but babies do not naturally fear the wide variety of objects and events that evoke anxiety in older children and adults. According to the classical conditioning model, these fears develop when a neutral stimulus that is initially incapable of causing anxiety becomes paired or associated with stimuli that *are* capable of eliciting fear or anxiety. As a consequence of the stimuli being paired together over time, the initially neutral stimulus acquires the ability to elicit anxiety on its own. Perhaps the prototypic human example of how anxiety may be conditioned is the classic case of the boy affectionately known in psychology texts as Little Albert (Watson & Rayner, 1920). John Watson and colleague tested Albert and found him to be unafraid of both live animals and various objects, such as cotton and burning newspaper. Albert did, not surprisingly, appear to become afraid when startled by a loud clanging sound produced by striking a steel bar with a hammer behind his back. The researchers then conditioned Albert to fear a white rat, which the boy was initially unafraid of, by banging loudly on the steel bar whenever Albert tried to touch the animal. Later, Albert began to react fearfully whenever the rat was present, even though Watson no longer banged on the bar. Albert also showed signs of being afraid of other stimuli that resembled the rat, such as a rabbit (a process called stimulus generalization).

Since the time of Watson, much research has demonstrated that fears may be conditioned and unconditioned in such a fashion in both humans and animals (see Bandura, 1969; Wolpe, 1973). Although classical conditioning was originally conceived of in behavioristic, nonmentalistic terms, there is growing agreement that conditioning of this nature is mediated by cognitive processes (Bandura, 1969; Goldfried, 1979; Murray & Jacobsen, 1971; Schwartz, 1982). Bandura (1969, p. 590) concludes that, "Rather than representing a simple process in which external stimuli are directly and automatically connected to overt responses, classical conditioning is partly mediated through symbolic activities." According to this view, the conditioned stimulus elicits cognitive activities that in turn produce autonomic responses, such as anxiety.

Extending classical conditioning to the realm of social anxiety, it is easy to see how negative experiences in social settings may condition a person to become anxious in similar situations in the future. Although a person may not have regarded certain social settings as unpleasant or anxiety-arousing at some earlier time, he or she now responds to such encounters as threatening because of previous aversive experiences. Although no studies have attempted to condition social anxiety in this manner (for obvious ethical reasons), many people are able to trace their social apprehensions to a specific incident in which they had an aversive social experience (Zimbardo, 1977). Imagine a teenage boy who is publicly ridiculed by a girl after he asks her to dance ("Can you imagine *he* wants to dance with *me*?"). It would not be surprising to learn that the boy faced future interactions with females with a bit of trepidation. Similarly, a woman may never have been anxious about speaking in public, but develop chronic audience anxiousness after bumbling her way through a particular travesty of a speech.

TREATMENT BASED ON CLASSICAL CONDITIONING

It follows from the classical conditioning approach that any response that was classically conditioned is potentially unconditionable through the same general process operating in reverse. Whereas anxiety was initially conditioned when aversive stimuli were associated with certain social settings or kinds of people, it may be deconditioned by pairing the aversive stimuli with factors that elicit more positive responses. If a response that inhibits anxiety, such as relaxation, can be evoked in the presence of the stimulus that causes the person to feel anxious, the conditioned bond will be weakened (Wolpe, 1973). This principle suggests that people can be conditioned to experience other responses in reaction to objects and events that currently make them nervous.

Therapists who adopt a conditioned anxiety approach to social anxiety typically use a variation of systematic desensitization as the treatment of choice for clients who are bothered by high social anxiousness. Although there are a number of variations, most desensitization regimens follow a relatively standard sequence. First, the client is trained in deep muscle relaxation (Jacobsen, 1938). Over a number of counseling sessions, the therapist teaches the anxious client how to relax his or her major muscle groups more or less at will. Through relaxation training, clients learn to relax far beyond the point at which most people are able to relax. The therapist and client then work together to construct an anxiety hierarchy, which is a list of the objects and events that make the client anxious, arranged according to the degree of anxiety elicited by each. Of course, each person has his or her personal list of anxiety-producing stimuli and may rank them in a different order than other people. In the case of social anxiousness, an anxiety hierarchy may include situations such as interacting in a small group, talking to someone of the other sex, talking to a stranger, giving a speech to a small audience, being the center of attention of a large group, and giving a speech to a large audience.

Once the client learns to relax on command and the hierarchy is developed, the therapist asks the client to relax and vividly imagine the least anxiety-producing event on the list. Whenever the client begins to feel nervous from thinking about the situation, he or she is told to stop imagining the scene until fully relaxed, then try again. (Some therapists encourage clients to continue to imagine the threatening scene and to try to cope with it; see Goldfried, 1980). After a while, the client is typically able to imagine the scene while remaining relaxed. With that accomplished, the client is asked to imagine the next event on the anxiety hierarchy. Again, the imagery may arouse anxiety, but with continued deep relaxation, the image of the situation loses its ability to elicit anxiety. Then, the third event on the hierarchy is imagined until it no longer evokes anxiety, and so on. Over a number of sessions, the client's social anxiousness typically decreases. The therapist and client must then work to assure that the newly acquired relaxation response generalizes to real life encounters. There are several procedures designed to facilitate in vivo generalization (Wolpe, 1973).

As originally conceived, the effectiveness of systematic desensitization was explained in terms of learning principles (Wolpe,

1958). However, more recently, cognitively oriented therapists have suggested that desensitization is effective because it gives clients a sense of control over their reactions to the feared object or event (Goldfried, 1980). It has also been found that cognitive rehearsal alone—imagining the anxiety-producing scenes without relaxation training—is sometimes effective in reducing anxiety (Folkins, Lawson, Opton, & Lazarus, 1968; Wilkins, 1971). Reconstrual of classical conditioning as a cognitive process has been accompanied by parallel changes in theoretical discussions of systematic desensitization.

In one of the earliest demonstrations of the efficacy of systematic desensitization for reduction of socially based anxieties, Paul (1966) assigned highly speech anxious subjects to one of four treatment groups. One group underwent a standard desensitization procedure similar to that described above. A second group received insight-oriented therapy; a third received a placebo pill and were told that it would reduce their speech anxiety; and a fourth, a no-treatment control group, participated in a public speaking course but received no counseling intervention. After six weeks, self-report, physiological, and behavioral indices of speech anxiety were taken. Although all three treatment groups, including the placebo subjects, showed a decrease on measures of public speaking anxiety, relative to the control group, subjects receiving systematic desensitization showed the greatest improvement on all measures of anxiety. (Interestingly, the five therapists used in the study favored insight-oriented treatments for speech anxiousness.) Follow-up data showed that the group who received-systematic desensitization scored lower on measures of speech anxiety than the other two treatment groups after two years (Paul, 1968).

Since Paul's groundbreaking research, dozens of other studies have shown that relative to no-treatment controls systematic desensitization is effective in reducing social anxiety in both children and adults (Bander, Steinke, Allen, & Mosher, 1975; Bandura, 1969; Curran, 1975; Curran & Gilbert, 1975; Fishman & Nawas, 1973; Kanter & Goldfried, 1979; Kirsch & Henry, 1979; Kondas, 1967; McCroskey, Richmond, Berger, & Baldwin, 1982; Meichenbaum, Gilmore, & Fedoravicius, 1971; Mitchell & Orr, 1974; O'Brien & Borkovec, 1977; Paul & Shannon, 1966). Kirsch and Henry (1979) have also demonstrated that self-administered systematic desensitization, in which clients learn the procedure from an instruction manual without direct intervention by a therapist, is effective in reducing speech anxiousness. Tape-recorded instructions are also effective (Goldfried & Davison, 1976). An off-shoot of systematic desensitization known as cue-controlled relaxation has been shown to be effective in the reduction of music performance anxiety among university music majors (Sweeney & Horan, 1982).[1]

CRITIQUE OF THE CONDITIONED ANXIETY MODEL

The conditioned anxiety approach has provided a useful perspective from which to understand and treat social anxiety. Although no studies have attempted to condition social anxiety in nonanxious people, research demonstrating the effectiveness of systematic desensitization in reducing social anxiousness supports the utility of the classical conditioning paradigm. However—and this point is often overlooked—the efficacy of systematic desensitization in reducing social anxiousness does not necessarily indicate that the individual's anxiety was initially classically conditioned. The cause and treatment of a condition do not bear any necessary logical relationship to one another. To use another example, we would not argue that the effectiveness of radiation therapy for certain forms of cancer demonstrates that the cancer developed because of insufficient radiation. In the same way, we cannot claim that the effectiveness of desensitization necessarily supports the conditioned anxiety model of social anxiety. I am not suggesting that social anxiety is not classically conditioned in many cases, only that we have no direct empirical evidence that it is.

Although the conditioned anxiety approach has been embraced by many counseling and clinical psychologists, as well as by practitioners in speech communication, it has hardly received more than a passing glance from personality and social psychologists. I see at least two possible reasons for this. First, most personality and social psychological research on social anxiety and related constructs has centered on either personality correlates of social anxiety or the interpersonal behaviors of socially anxious people. This emphasis on personological and behavioral aspects of social anxiety does not lead easily to an interest in the development or remediation of social anxiousness through classical conditioning. Another way of saying this is that the topics and paradigms of greatest interest to personality and social psychologists do not spring from a classical conditioning perspective.

A second reason for the lack of interest may be a misunderstanding among many personality and social psychologists regarding current thinking on classical conditioning. Viewing classical conditioning in traditional, noncognitive terms may have deterred researchers from adopting a conditioning model in an era characterized by an emphasis on social cognition (e.g., Higgins, Herman, & Zanna, 1980). However, as I noted earlier, classical conditioning may be encompassed within a cognitive framework so that the conditioning model of social anxiety is not necessarily incompatible with cognitive approaches. But, for whatever reason, work stemming from the conditioned anxiety model of social anxiety has emerged exclusively from counseling and clinical research on systematic desensitization.

Skills Deficit Approach

People differ widely in the degree to which they typically respond in ways that facilitate social interactions. We all know people who seem to have a knack for responding in a poised and skillful manner. Their responses are appropriate and well timed, they communicate clearly and effectively, and their forthrightness stimulates openness and honesty in others. At the other extreme, we also know people whom others regard as socially deficient in certain respects. These individuals may tend to respond inappropriately (if at all) to others, communicate ineffectively, display undesirable or annoying mannerisms, have difficulty holding up their end of conversations, and so on. Although the classification of particular behaviors as indicative of "good" versus "poor" social skills is a value-laden judgment, most of us can, at least intuitively, identify people we regard as socially adept and others we view as socially unskilled.

The social skills deficit approach posits that many instances of social anxiety are directly or indirectly the consequence of poor social skills. Since smooth and satisfying encounters with others require a minimal ability to interact in a socially skilled and facilitative manner, people who cannot do so are likely to create aversive social situations for themselves. The aversive consequences of poor social skills come from three main sources. First, the person who does not interact with at least a modicum of skill is likely to receive less than positive reactions from others. When an individual responds in a way that others regard as inappropriate, ineffective, or unskillful, they are likely to provide implicit or explicit feedback which the offending individual will perceive as disapproving or rejecting (Arkowitz et al., 1978).

Second, unskilled social reactions are likely to create an awkward situation for all participants. When someone responds inappropriately or has difficulty responding, the encounter is thrown off-track. The efforts of the interactants must then be directed toward remedying the situation so that normal interaction may resume. Thus, the individual who inadvertently mismanages his or her dealings with others on a regular basis is likely to experience a high proportion of awkward, stilted encounters that elicit feelings of anxiety. Third, the self-perception that one's social responses are not satisfactory may result in social anxiety. People monitor their behavior and evaluate its adequacy even without feedback from others. Thus, a man addressing a civic group may perceive that his talk is incomprehensible, his mannerisms stilted, and his speech disfluent even without feedback from the audience. The self-perception that one's social behaviors are lacking may trigger social anxiety.

The concept of social skill continues to be problematic for researchers in clinical and counseling psychology. As Curran (1979, p. 321) notes, "Everyone seems to know what good and poor skills are but no one can define them adequately." To go into the various conceptualizations of social skill and the problems associated with each would require much more room than we are able to devote to the topic here. The interested reader is referred to Bellack and Hersen (1979; especially the chapter by Curran), Libet and Lewinsohn (1972), and McFall (1982).

Rather than attempt a specific definition of social skill, I will point out three major classes of social skill deficits. First, people may not know how to execute a particular type of social response. For example, an individual may be unable to formulate a cogent compliment, express condolences, initiate sex, or tell interesting anecdotes. People who have not been exposed to socially skilled models may lack the cognitive representations necessary to reproduce such behaviors. Second, people may know in a technical sense *how* a particular social behavior should be performed and yet have problems with the specific details of its execution. Bellack (1979) notes that people may have problems with the frequency, duration, intensity, or form of a particular social response. For example, eye contact is an important component of face-to-face interactions since it indicates attentiveness to what others are saying, conveys certain emotional reactions, and provides cues that facilitate turn-taking during the conversation. Some individuals, however, may look at others too often or too infrequently (a frequency problem), look too briefly at each glance or for too prolonged a period of time (a duration problem), appear to look too intently or too casually (an intensity problem), or combine eye contact with other behaviors, such as touching, that obscure the meaning of the gaze (a problem involving the form of the response). In any of these cases, the person's gazing behavior is likely to be perceived by others as inappropriate (e.g., "He can't even look me in the eye when we talk."), create awkward moments during the conversation, lead some interactants to shun the individual as a conversationalist, and, as a result, cause the person who has problems with eye contact to feel socially anxious.

A third kind of social skill problem arises when people are actually capable of responding appropriately and skillfully, but are unable or unwilling to execute the needed behaviors. Most of us have, at times, held back from doing or saying the most socially appropriate or facilitative thing although we were quite capable of doing so in a skilled manner. A woman may know how to skillfully express a compliment or ask a man for a date, but have difficulty making herself do so because of potential social risks. Similarly, a college student may have profound ideas to contribute to class discussion and be capable of expressing them articulately yet fail to volunteer in class.

SKILL DIFFERENCES BETWEEN HIGH AND LOW SOCIALLY ANXIOUS PEOPLE

If the social skill deficit hypothesis is correct in its assumption that social anxiety results from skill deficits, we would expect to observe distinct differences in the social skill level of people who are classified as high versus low in social anxiousness. Presumably, people who are deficient in social skill experience greater difficulties in social encounters, receive less positive feedback from others, view themselves as less skilled, and experience social anxiety more often than people who interact more skillfully. An examination of studies that have examined differences between high and low socially anxious individuals reveals mixed findings.

On one hand, several studies have found that observers rate highly socially anxious people (identified on the basis of self-report measures) as generally less socially skilled than people who are low in social anxiousness (e.g., Arkowitz, Lichtenstein, McGovern, & Hines, 1975; Bellack & Hersen, 1979; Curran, 1977; Farrell, Mariotto, Conger, Curran, & Wallander, 1979; Monti, 1982; Twentyman & McFall, 1975). This finding has been replicated using a number of different kinds of observers (experimenters, trained raters, confederates, other naive subjects, friends) and a number of contexts (real-life interactions, role-playing exercises, videotapes of laboratory interactions, audiotapes of conversations). Although a few studies have not obtained differences (e.g., Clark & Arkowitz, 1975), most studies conclude that observers perceive socially anxious people to be less socially skilled.

However, studies that have sought *specific* skill differences (as opposed to observers' *ratings* of general social skill) have identified few behavioral differences between high and low socially anxious subjects, and it is not clear that these differences constitute differences in social *skill.* For example, compared to low anxious people, socially anxious subjects have been found to speak less in conversations, look less at other interactants, nod and smile more frequently, interrupt less often, and engage in more backchannel responding—the sounds people make to indicate they are listening to another, such as "uh-huh" (Arkowitz et al., 1975; Borkovec et al., 1974; Cheek & Buss, 1981; Leary, 1980; Natale, Entin, & Jaffe, 1979; Pilkonis, 1977b). Whether these findings are indicative of social skill differences is questionable. In fact, it could be argued that socially anxious people display *more* socially facilitative responses, such as greater attentiveness to other interactants. Perhaps highly socially anxious people are more skilled as "listeners," whereas less anxious people are more skilled as "speakers" in contingent interactions.

These behavioral data are quite inconsistent with the observers' ratings described earlier: Observers report that socially anxious people are low in social skill, but repeated attempts to identify skill differences have come up empty-handed. There are a number of possible reasons for this apparent discrepancy. First, few of the behaviors examined in these studies are actually indicative of social skill level. For example, a low level of social participation does not, in itself, indicate poor social skills. In fact, a *high* level of participation may be socially disruptive, as in the case of the overly talkative boor who does not realize his or her adverse impact upon others. Similarly, neither a low nor a high amount of eye contact is necessarily appropriate in all instances; either too much or too little eye contact may be problematic. Future research should focus on behaviors that are more clearly indicative of social skill, such as making clearly inappropriate comments, failing to respond adequately to others' queries, and communicating ineffectively. The available behavioral data simply do not adequately address the question of social skill differences between high and low socially anxious people.

Related to this, Fischetti, Curran, and Wessberg (1977) suggested that the skill deficits that are related to social anxiety are not reflected in the simple behaviors that have been studied, such as frequency of eye contact and the proportion of time spent talking in a conversation. These kinds of measures ignore the reciprocal nature of contingent encounters. Effective social participation requires that interactants tailor their responses to the ongoing encounter as well as to the context in which it occurs and time their contributions appropriately. Fischetti et al. (1977) proposed that high and low socially anxious people might differ more in the *timing and placement* of their responses than in the frequency or duration of them.

In an ingeneous test of this hypothesis, Fischetti et al. told male subjects that they would be listening to a female talk about herself over an intercom. Subjects were to respond to what she was saying by pressing a switch at those points in the conversation at which they would normally make a verbal or gestural response such as saying "uh-huh" or nodding. Depressing the switch would ostensibly activate a light that the woman would see. Subjects then listened to a prerecorded tape of a woman talking about herself while researchers recorded the placement of their responses to her. Results showed that low skill-high anxiety and high skill-low axiety men did not differ in the *number* of times they responded to the woman's remarks by pressing the switch. However, they differed greatly in the timing and placement of their responses. The responses of high skill-low anxiety men tended to cluster around a number of discrete "popular intervals" in the woman's monologue, points at which a high percentage of subjects responded. If you'll think about listening to someone talk during a conversation, it is easy to see that there are certain points at which responses by the listener are more appropriate than others. Apparently, the highly socially skilled men recognized these appropriate points and confined most of their responses to them.

The researchers were unable to identify any popular intervals in the responses of the low skill-high anxiety subjects, however. These men were no more likely to respond at specific points than at others, strewing their responses, more or less, randomly throughout the conversation! Fischetti et al. conclude that the low skill-high anxiety subjects lacked clear guidelines regarding the appropriate places to respond during a conversation.[2]

Another explanation of the lack of congruence between observers' subjective ratings and the objective behavioral measures is that observers may partially base their assessment of a person's social skill on overt manifestations of nervousness. That is, appearing nervous may connote low social skill. If this is the case, highly socially anxious people would, quite naturally, be perceived as less skilled.

A final possible explanation is that different people have different skill deficits. The failure to detect objective behavioral skill differences between low and high socially anxious individuals only shows that the two groups do not differ systematically on a particular behavior. If each socially anxious individual has a relatively idiosyncratic pattern of behavioral difficulties, skill differences would be detected by observers but not be revealed in analyses of specific behaviors.

To summarize this section: Socially anxious people are regarded by others as less socially skilled than less anxious people, providing some support for the social skills deficit approach. However, the precise nature of these skill deficits has not been determined.

SOCIAL SKILLS TRAINING

Operating under the assumption that many people experience social difficulties because of poor social skills, many therapists adopt a skills training model for clients who are bothered by chronically high social anxiousness (for reviews see Bellack & Hersen, 1979; Curran, 1977; Glaser, 1981). Although the specific procedures used differ from study to study, most research has shown that social skills training reduces socially anxious subjects' anxiety (Bellack & Hersen, 1979; Curran, 1975, 1977; Curran & Gilbert, 1975; Curran, Gilbert, & Little, 1976; Fremouw & Zitter, 1978; Glass et al., 1976; MacDonald, Lindquist, Kramer, McGrath, & Rhyne, 1975). In most studies, social skills training has been found to be as effective as alternative treatments in reducing anxiety, but, not surprisingly, more effective than other procedures in improving social skills.

There are two general approaches to skills remediation. The choice between them depends upon whether the client appears to possess adequate skills but has difficulty actually executing them, or whether the client actually lacks important social skills. In cases in which the anxious client appears not to possess a repertoire of socially skilled responses, a "response acquisition" approach is typically used (Bandura, 1969). Put simply, the client learns new social responses. The particular social behaviors that are targeted for remediation depend to a degree upon the specific nature of the client's difficulties as assessed by the counselor. Once problem areas are identified, a number of procedures are employed to teach the client more facilitative ways of interacting. Typically, the client observes socially skilled models, receives explicit instruction about how best to respond, role-plays certain skilled behaviors (i.e., behavioral rehearsal), observes and evaluates his or her behavior on videotape, and receives feedback and reinforcement from the counselor. In many instances, clients practice their newly learned ways of interacting on the therapist, assistants, or other clients, and do regular "homework" assignments in which they use the skills in real life encounters. These attempts are discussed at the next meeting with the counselor and additional exercises involving that skill are completed if necessary. In short, skill acquisition is similar to learning any set of complex responses.

In other instances, the counselor may perceive that the client understands how to respond in a skilled, facilitative manner but has difficulty actually doing so, often because of a lack of experience or self-confidence in a particular social domain. In these cases, a "response practice" model is often used. Clients are given the opportunity to practice appropriate social behaviors in relatively nonthreatening settings. For example, some counselors arrange interactions and/or practice dates between socially anxious men and women. Outcome studies show that practice alone, even without teaching or coaching by a therapist, is effective in reducing social anxiousness in many cases (Arkowitz et al., 1978; Bander et al., 1975; Christensen & Arkowitz, 1974; Martinson &

Zerface, 1970). It is not clear, however, whether the effectiveness of "response practice" is due to improving social skills, to increased confidence in one's ability to handle certain social encounters, to in vivo desensitization (Royce & Arkowitz, 1978), or to some other factor. In addition, certain weaknesses in the designs of many of these studies obscure their results (see Curran, in press).

Since the response practice approach to social anxiety is a highly efficient way of reducing some clients' social anxiousness (since it requires minimal time with a professional), its effectiveness should be more adequately assessed. If response practice is conclusively shown to reduce social anxiousness, we must find a way to identify those clients who would benefit most from it—namely those who have good social skills but who need experience using them. In addition, research is needed that assesses the utility of response acquisition and response practice approaches for reducing various manifestations of audience anxiousness. Most research in the area has focused on the reduction of social anxiety in contingent, usually heterosexual interactions.

CRITIQUE OF THE SKILLS DEFICIT APPROACH

There is little doubt that a link exists between social skills and social anxiety but the precise nature of this relationship is not clear. First, social skill difficulties are neither a necessary nor sufficient precondition for the experience of social anxiety. Many people who experience a high level of social anxiety are actually quite socially adept. Curran and Gilbert (1975, p. 520) observed one female in their sample who "was so concerned about her social ability that she would become nauseous before a date; yet, subjectively she appeared to her group leaders to be highly skilled." Zimbardo (1977) reports the cases of many celebrities, such as Johnny Carson and Barbara Walters, who say that they often feel shy. These individuals would seem to be anything but low in social skill.[3] The social skills model is not able to explain why highly skilled people are often highly socially anxious.

Nor is the approach able to account for people who are, by everyone else's standards, bumbling, boring, socially incompetent individuals but who appear to experience social anxiety only rarely. Why are all socially unskilled people not highly socially anxious?

The social skills deficit hypothesis is easily salvaged if we focus on people's *beliefs* about their own social behaviors rather than on their actual behaviors. The revised hypothesis is that people become socially anxious when they believe that they are behaving in a socially unskilled fashion. When considered in terms of individuals' subjective perceptions of their social skill, the skills deficit model may be subsumed by a broader perspective that focuses on cognitive mediators of social anxiety.

The Cognitive Approaches

It would be misleading to suggest that there is a "cognitive theory" of social anxiety. Cognitive approaches to social anxiety constitute a loose grouping of hypotheses regarding ways in which people's beliefs about themselves and about their social worlds precipitate feelings of social anxiety. As such, they represent several of the growing number of cognitive models of psychological phenomena, models that have already been applied to topics as diverse as motivation, depression, and stress. Although a number of cognitive approaches to social anxiety have been proposed, these may be loosely grouped into three categories.

NEGATIVE SELF-EVALUATIONS

The negative self-evaluation variation of the cognitive approach hypothesizes that people become socially anxious when they evaluate themselves unfavorably on important social dimensions. When people regard themselves negatively and/or believe they will be unable to handle the social demands of a particular encounter, they are likely to experience social anxiety (Clark & Arkowitz, 1975; Meichenbaum et al., 1971; Rehm & Marston, 1968). Viewed from this perspective, whether their negative self-evaluations are warranted is beside the point. Imagined social deficiencies are as likely to trigger social anxiety as real ones. This point helps explain why data reflecting upon the social skills hypothesis are equivocal.

According to the negative self-evaluation model, the self-perception of skill deficits is of greater importance in precipitating social anxiety than are actual skill deficits per se. Since people often misperceive their true level of social skill, actual skill level and social anxiety are poorly correlated.

Two lines of research support the self-evaluation conceptualization of social anxiety. First, several studies have obtained moderately strong negative correlations (in the vicinity of $-.50$ in most cases) between measures of self-evaluation, notably self-esteem, and self-report measures of social anxiety (Cheek, 1982; Leary, 1983a; Leavy, 1980), social avoidance and distress (Clark & Arkowitz, 1975), shyness (Cheek & Buss, 1981; Zimbardo, 1977), and communication apprehension (Huntley, 1969; McCroskey, 1975, 1977). Thus, evaluating oneself unfavorably is associated with higher than average social anxiousness. In a similar vein, people who are low in self-esteem report experiencing significantly greater anxiety in laboratory interactions than high self-esteem people (Leavy, 1980).

A second set of studies has shown that socially anxious people generate a greater number of negative self-statements before and during interpersonal encounters. That is, when asked to report what they are thinking, socially anxious individuals say they are thinking about how poorly they expect to perform in the encounter, how negatively they are likely to be evaluated by other interactants, and that they are pondering their social deficiencies (Cacioppo, Glass, & Merluzzi, 1979; Clark & Arkowitz, 1975; Glass, Merluzzi, Biever, & Larsen, 1982). There is no way to show that these sorts of self-thoughts actually *cause* social anxiety, but an association between self-derogation and nervousness in social encounters is undisputed.

The social difficulties of low self-esteem people are exacerbated by the fact that people remember information about themselves more easily when it is consistent with their self-schema (Markus, 1980). Research on memory for self-relevent information suggests that once people view themselves and their social performances negatively, they are more likely to recall incidents in which they performed poorly rather than skillfully and more likely to remember unfavorable than favorable reactions from others. As a result, these easily accessed negative memories serve to precipitate social anxiety when future encounters are contemplated.

In the only study of this effect, O'Banion and Arkowitz (1977) classified women as either low or high in social anxiousness on the basis of the Social Avoidance and Distress Scale (Watson & Friend, 1969). The women interacted with a male confederate for seven minutes, then received an adjective checklist upon which the male had ostensibly indicated his impression of them. (These ratings were actually contrived by the researchers to reflect a mix of positive and negative attributes.) After viewing the rating, subjects were asked which of another list of 80 adjectives had been checked by the male with whom they had interacted. In essence, they were asked to recall the male's rating of them. Consistent with previous research on memory, highly socially anxious women remembered a significantly higher number of the negative adjectives than the less anxious women. Apparently, their negative self-schema biased their recall of the male's ratings in the direction of less flattering traits. The tendency to recall information more easily when it is consistent with self-schema may be one reason that negative self-evaluations are so difficult to change.

IRRATIONAL BELIEFS

A second set of cognitions that have been hypothesized to promote social anxiety includes so-called irrational beliefs about the importance of being liked by others. As Ellis (1962) proposed, many individuals believe that it is important for them to be loved and approved of by virtually everyone and that less than full acceptance by others is indicative of failure and unworthiness as a person. Ellis designated these beliefs as "irrational" because they constitute unattainable goals and ultimately result in insecurity and unhappiness rather than security, happiness, and personal adjustment. According to this perspective, people who place an undue emphasis on universal social approval tend to feel insecure and socially anxious when dealing with others since they never achieve the full acceptance they desire.

Goldfried and Sobocinski (1975) administered the Irrational Beliefs Test (Jones, 1968) and two measures of social anxiousness to 77 undergraduate women. The Irrational Beliefs Test measures the degree of respondents' endorsement of the 10 irrational beliefs identified by Ellis, including the irrational demand for approval described above. As predicted by this version of the cognitive approach to social anxiety, an overemphasis on gaining others' acceptance was positively correlated with scores on the Social Avoidance and Distress Scale ($r = .36$, $p < .01$) and the Personal Report of Confidence as a Speaker ($r = .33$, $p < .01$). Apparently, social anxiousness is related specifically to this particular irrational belief rather than to irrational beliefs in general: Glass et al. (1982) failed to obtain a difference between high and low socially anxious females' total scores on the Irrational Beliefs Test.

EXCESSIVELY HIGH STANDARDS

People who hold excessively high standards for evaluating their own social behaviors and outcomes are, like those who desire approval from everyone, likely to consistently fall short of their goals. The third cognitive approach to social anxiety suggests that social anxiety sometimes results from unrealistically high standards. As Bandura (1969, p. 37) observed, many people who seek professional help for anxiety "are neither incompetent nor anxiously inhibited, but they experience a great deal of personal distress stemming from excessively high standards for self-evaluation, often supported by unfavorable comparisons with models noted for their extraordinary achievements." Research on this hypothesis is sparse. However, consistent with this view, people who hold unrealistically high expectations for themselves tend to score higher on the Social Avoidance and Distress Scale ($r = .55$, $p < .001$) and the Personal Report of Confidence as a Speaker ($r = .37$, $p < .001$; Goldfried & Sobocinski, 1975).

COGNITIVE-BASED TREATMENTS FOR SOCIAL ANXIOUSNESS

Since all three cognitive approaches assume that social anxiety is cognitively mediated, it is not surprising that their proponents recommend cognitive treatments for social anxiousness—treatments that focus on modifying people's beliefs about themselves and their social relationships. A number of cognitive therapies have appeared in the last decade, all of them having in common an emphasis on the role of cognition in determining affect and behavior. Although a detailed examination of these approaches would take us far afield, we will briefly describe the general approach. The interested reader is referred to Meichenbaum (1977) for a seminal treatment of cognitive therapy.

Two different lines of work have converged to create contemporary cognitive therapy, one stemming from Ellis' (1962) emphasis on irrational beliefs and the other growing from Meichenbaum's (1977) attention to self-verbalizations and cognitive-behavior modification. Although these two models have different lineages, most cognitively oriented therapists borrow freely from both. In the prototypic cognitive therapy (such as cognitive modification or rational restructuring), socially anxious clients are first taught that their high level of anxiety is a product of their thoughts about themselves and about social encounters. The role of irrational beliefs including high expectations and/or negative, self-defeating self-thoughts in precipitating anxiety is emphasized. They are then taught to recognize irrational thoughts and negative self-thoughts as they arise and to substitute more adaptive cognitions. Clients with irrational beliefs are led to appraise social encounters and their performance in them more objectively (e.g., "Will it really be so awful if I don't make a good impression on her?"), whereas those who tend to self-deprecate are taught to substitute more positive and realistic self-thoughts for their typically negative ones (e.g., "I'll probably do just fine during our date tonight, so why worry?"). In short, socially anxious clients are taught new ways of viewing themselves and their relationships with others that facilitate their ability to cope with socially stressful situations.

A great deal of counseling research has demonstrated the effectiveness of cognitive therapy in reducing anxiety experienced in a variety of social contexts (Fremouw & Zitter, 1978; Glass et al., 1976; Kanter & Goldfried, 1979; Malkiewich & Merluzzi, 1980; Meichenbaum et al., 1971; Rehm & Marston, 1968; Sanchez-Craig,

1976). Cognitive restructuring is also effective in reducing musical performance anxiety—an underresearched manifestation of social anxiety (Sweeney & Horan, 1982). Cognitively based therapies have consistently proven as effective as skills training and desensitization in reducing social anxiousness and occasionally are more effective. Cognitive therapies seem to have the advantage of generalizing more easily to new social and nonsocial situations than skills training and desensitization, which tend to focus on difficulties experienced in specific kinds of social settings (Glass et al., 1976; Kanter & Goldfried, 1979; see, however, Fremouw & Zitter, 1978). For detailed reviews of the literature regarding cognitive therapies, see Goldfried (1979) and Glaser (1981).

Haemmerlie and Montgomery (1982) have recently advocated an alternative method of modifying clients' unfavorable evaluations of their ability to interact successfully with others. Based upon Bem's self-perception theory (1972) they reasoned that anxious clients' negative self-perceptions may be modified by unobtrusively leading them to believe that they had performed competently in a series of social situations. Over a series of positive encounters, clients would come to view themselves and their social abilities more favorably, thus reducing their social anxiousness. In a study designed to test this hypothesis, socially anxious males interacted with six different female confederates (who subjects believed were naive subjects like themselves) for 12 minutes each. The confederates were instructed to respond as positively as possible during the conversations, thus providing the men with six seemingly independent sources of positive social feedback. Results showed that subjects who were exposed to this procedure became less socially anxious and more self-confident, subsequently initiated more conversations with women, and were more open about themselves in another cross-sex conversation. These changes were maintained up to six months, during which time these men also showed an increase in the frequency with which they dated. The impact of these short, unobtrusively biased interactions with six members of the other sex was surprisingly strong, and implicates the lack of positive social feedback as an antecedent of low self-esteem and social anxiousness.

Future research is needed on this approach since it appears to be a very cost-effective way of reducing some cases of heterosocial anxiousness. In particular, we need to know whether the obtained effects are due to simple social skill practice (e.g., Christensen, Arkowitz, & Anderson, 1975), to desensitization (since the encounters were pleasant and nonthreatening), to increased feelings of self-efficacy (Bandura, 1977), to improved evaluations of oneself, or, more likely, to some combination of these factors.

CRITIQUE OF THE COGNITIVE APPROACHES

Despite the demonstrated effectiveness of cognitive therapies and the data supporting the cognitive mediation of social anxiety, several questions regarding these treatments and their theoretical underpinnings have not been adequately addressed. First, research on the effectiveness of cognitive therapies has often included specific behavioral and anxiety-reduction procedures within the cognitive treatment conditions. Thus, in many studies, purely cognitive approaches to therapy are confounded by techniques derived from other models. In a practical sense, this is all right since cognitive and noncognitive approaches are often combined in treatments used by practitioners who deal with socially anxious clients. However, confounded experimental manipulations do not allow us to assess the relative contributions of cognitive modifications compared to other treatments. Similarly, cognitive therapies themselves include a number of relatively discrete components, such as insight into the role of cognition in anxiety, identification of negative self-statements, and the learning of coping responses. Component analyses of cognitive treatments for social anxiousness are needed to examine the relative contributions of each component to the therapeutic effect. One such study suggests that all major components of the treatment are necessary for maximum effectiveness (Glogower, Fremouw, & McCroskey, 1978).

A second methodological weakness that leaves important questions unanswered is that few studies of cognitive treatment of social anxiousness have included measures of *cognitive* change (e.g., Kanter & Goldfried, 1979). Glass et al. (1982) argue that we should not infer that the effectiveness of cognitive therapies lies in the modification of clients' cognitions unless we have direct evidence of cognitive change. Future research should include measures of subject-clients' cognitions, such as the Social Interaction Self-Statement Test (Glass et al., 1982) or unstructured thought-listing procedures (Cacioppo et al., 1980).

A third treatment-related question is whether changes in clients' cognitions and level of social anxiousness are accompanied by behavioral changes. Presumably, more positive views of oneself and more adaptive, "rational" thoughts about social interaction would be accompanied by a greater willingness to participate in previously threatening encounters. At present, the research findings on this question are equivocal (see Glass et al., 1976; Kanter & Goldfried, 1979).

Despite lingering questions, it seems to me that of the three perspectives discussed in this chapter the cognitive approaches do the best job of accounting for social anxiety and for treatment effects. Not only do the cognitive approaches account for a great deal of data, they also appear to subsume both the classical conditioning and social skill models. Inasmuch as current explanations of classical conditioning emphasize the role of cognitive processes, conditioning may be easily incorporated into a broader cognitive approach to social anxiety. In the same way, the cognitive perspective easily subsumes the skills deficit approach by hypothesizing that people feel socially anxious when they *believe* they lack important social skills.

This latter point is nicely demonstrated by a recent study that identified two distinct kinds of people who experience social anxiety when interacting with those of the other sex. Curran, Wallander, and Fischetti (1980) found that some socially anxious subjects had clear-cut skill deficits and accurately recognized their own social limitations. These people had social difficulties, knew it, and consequently felt socially anxious. Other socially anxious subjects showed evidence of *good* social skills, but yet they too were highly anxious. Why? The data supported a cognitive interpretation. The high skill-high anxiety subjects *underestimated* their level of social ability, compared to judges' ratings. Curran et al. suggest that the distinction between these two groups of socially anxious people is of clinical importance since they actually have very different kinds of social difficulties. I will return to this point in a later chapter.

The cognitive approaches also explain why some people who are clearly lacking in interpersonal skill *do not* feel socially anxious. Viewed from the cognitive perspective, such individuals either do not recognize their social limitations or do not place great importance upon them.

Although the cognitive approaches we have been discussing do the best job of single-handedly explaining social anxiety of the models discussed so far, they leave a few important questions unanswered. First, negative self-evaluations do not always cause people to experience social anxiety. Most people realistically recognize that they are below average in certain social and nonsocial respects. Some people know they cannot tell a joke well, others know that people do not regard them as attractive, some know they have difficulty being an interesting conversationalist, and so on. Yet, most of these individuals go through their everyday lives with only minimal social anxiety. Their feelings of social insecurity are triggered only in certain social settings and when dealing with certain kinds of people. The cognitive approach does not specify the conditions under which negative self-evaluations and irrational beliefs will and will not precipitate social anxiety.

On the other hand, people sometimes feel socially anxious even though they evaluate themselves quite highly and hold no unrealistic expectations—an observation that current cognitive approaches have difficulty explaining. A man may think he performed superbly on a job interview, or played his part well in a play, or was as charming as one could be on a date, but may still feel anxious. Why? As we will see in the next chapter, the answer appears to have something to do with the distinction between his *self-evaluation and how he thinks others* will evaluate him. In each example above, the man may believe that relevant others (the interviewer, theatre critics, his date) were not suitably impressed despite his strong performance in each instance. It may be that the central factor in social anxiety is not self-evaluation per se, but concerns about evaluations by others.

Notes

1. In a recent development, McCroskey et al. (1982) present evidence that the efficacy of systematic desensitization for reducing communication apprehension is *decreased* when the procedure is paired with public speaking courses and/or speaking skills training. Although the meta-analyses underlying this conclusion may be questioned and a cogent explanation for such a finding is difficult to formulate, this possibility is intriguing and invites an empirical test within a single study.

2. This study has subsequently been replicated using female subjects, with virtually identical results (Peterson, Fischetti, Curran, & Arland, 1981).

3. Several of my colleagues are unable to believe that the seemingly poised and extraverted celebrities who claim to be "shy" actually have social difficulties. Although we can not discount the possibility that some people claim to be "shy" because it connotes reserve and modesty, it is indeed possible for extraverted people to be socially anxious. As we will see in a later chapter, some people are able to be quite extraverted and sociable in spite of a high level of subjective anxiety.

3

SELF-PRESENTATION AND SOCIAL ANXIETY

As we saw in the last chapter, each of the three major theoretical perspectives contributes to our understanding of social anxiety but none is fully adequate to explain all instances in which people become socially anxious. In this chapter we will examine a social psychological theory of social anxiety that Barry Schlenker and I have developed over the past few years (Leary, 1980, 1982; Leary & Schlenker, 1981; Schlenker & Leary, 1982). As will become clear in subsequent chapters, this approach has four advantages over the three perspectives just discussed: It specifies within a single theory the necessary and sufficient conditions for all instances in which people feel socially anxious; it makes clear predictions regarding situational and dispositional factors that should be associated with high social anxiety; it is consistent with virtually all existing data in the area; and it provides a framework for making *client-specific* recommendations for the treatment of high social anxiousness. Before turning to the theory itself, it is necessary to set the stage by reviewing a few basic social psychological principles.

Social Exchange and Interpersonal Behavior

Nearly all of the outcomes that people strive to attain in life are mediated by other people. Whatever people desire, it is unlikely that they will obtain it without dealing with others. Whether people need material goods (such as food, clothing, or personal belongings) or social commodities (such as friendship, love, acceptance, or security), they are usually dependent upon others to help fulfill their needs and wants. Similarly, many negative events in life, such as rejection, monetary fines, a denied promotion, physical punishment, and public humiliation, occur because of the actions of other people. Because people's lives are highly interdependent, one can think of few outcomes in life that don't involve others in one way or another.

However, valued physical and social commodities in life are not free for the taking. People do not typically receive positive outcomes from others unless they have "earned" them in some respect. Others do not generally give us affection, respect, promotions, standing ovations, compliments, and other social rewards for absolutely no reason. Similarly, whether we like to admit it or not, a high proportion of the *negative* outcomes we receive from others are justly deserved. Since the positive and negative outcomes people receive are partially dependent upon the actions of others, it is usually in their best interests to influence others directly or indirectly to respond to them in personally satisfying ways.

The individual's effect upon others' treatment of him or her provides the basis of social exchange theory (Homans, 1974; Thibaut & Kelley, 1959). According to this approach to human interaction, people exchange social commodities for those they desire from others much in the same way that people exchange money for goods and services in the marketplace. The adage, "To have a friend, be a friend," illustrates the idea of social exchange. Since you are unlikely to be my friend and treat me well if I give nothing in return, I will exchange my friendship, assistance, and good will for yours, and we will both end up with positive social outcomes. At the same time, my expressions of friendship will help forestall malicious behavior on your part, and vice versa. I can influence, to a degree, how you will respond to me by treating you in certain ways.

Buss (1983) distinguishes between two major types of rewards people receive from others, which he calls economic and social. According to Buss, economic rewards are those that must be earned, bought, or bartered, such as money, goods, and services.

Social rewards, such as praise, status, and love, need not be earned according to Buss but are freely exchanged among close friends and family. Although this distinction has merit in some contexts, it obscures the fact that even social rewards are generally not heaped upon the recipient without cause. Even among friends and family, we normally do not lavish praise, respect, or affection upon those who are, in our eyes, undeserving of such treatment. Of course, close friends and family may dispense both economic and social rewards more freely than do total strangers, but even then rewards are not given indiscriminately.

It should be emphasized that social outcomes are not necessarily exchanged "tit-for-tat" on a commodity by commodity basis. The social rules of exchange differ depending upon the nature of the relationship between the two individuals (Mills & Clark, 1982). In an "exchange relationship," individuals adhere to a rule that says that the receipt of a benefit from the other should be "repaid" sooner or later by the giving of a benefit of comparable value. If a colleague buys you lunch today, it is likely that you will return a similar favor sometime in the future. In a "communal relationship," however, people operate under the assumption that the receipt of a benefit does not incur a debt. Rather, because each member of a communal relationship is interested in the well-being of the other, positive outcomes are given and received without the expectation of "repayment" on either side. In a close friendship or romantic relationship, for example, benefits are freely given and received with little concern for tit-for-tat exchange. Even so, if over time one member of the relationship believes that he or she is giving more than is being received, feelings of inequity will result (e.g., Walster, Walster, & Berscheid, 1978).

This view of human interactions and relationships, phrased in terms of exchange and influence, often strikes people as degrading and cynical, bringing to mind images of manipulative self-seekers attempting to trick or coerce others to do their bidding. However, social influence in everyday encounters and relationships is neither consciously manipulative nor coercive. Only the very powerful enjoy the prerogative of forcibly inducing others' compliance, and even they can't force others to give them valued social outcomes, such as friendship, affection, and respect (although they may get others to *act* in such ways). It is because most of us have no direct power to control others' treatment of us that we rely upon the principles of social exchange in an attempt to bring about the social outcomes we desire. A man may want his date to like him, a friend to vote for a particular political candidate, or his boss to recommend him for a promotion. But he can acquire these outcomes only by influencing others, intentionally or unintentionally, to respond as he wishes. He must "earn" affection from his date by being a likeable fellow, he must persuade his friend via convincing arguments, and he must demonstrate to his boss that he is worthy of the promotion. In each case, the desired outcomes are acquired through a subtle social exchange and influence process.

Self-Presentation

Given that most social and material rewards and punishments come at the hands of others, it is not surprising that people want to influence others to treat them in personally desirable ways. Among the ways in which people try to influence others' treatment of them is *self-presentation,* sometimes called impression management. Self-presentation is the attempt to control the self-relevent images one projects to others (Schlenker, 1980).

When people deal with others, they respond in part on the basis of the *impressions* they have formed. During interpersonal encounters, people obtain many pieces of information about others from a variety of sources, gleaning information from their appearance, speech, actions, nonverbal behaviors, reputation, and so on. They then process and combine these data to form an overall impression of what the person is like (Schlenker, 1980). This impression contains both the information that was actually observed (the person's appearance or occupation, for example) and inferences about the person based upon the observed attributes (such as inferences about the person's attitudes, motives, or values). The impressions people form of others often go far beyond what was actually observed.

Once people have formed impressions of others, their behavior toward them is strongly affected by those impressions. If people have formed a positive, favorable impression of an individual—that she is kind, honest, and humorous, for example—they are likely to react positively toward her. They will probably like her, be nice to her, compliment her, help her in times of trouble, and offer any number of other social and/or material rewards. On the other hand, if they have formed a negative, unfavorable impression of the person, whether accurate or not, they are likely to respond in ways that she considers undesirable. If they see her as selfish, unfriendly, and dogmatic, for example, they are likely to criticize her, react coldly in her presence, refuse to socialize with her, not recommend her for raises, promotions, honors, or special assignments, sabotage her efforts, and so on. In short, interpersonal encounters and the process of social exchange are strongly affected by the nature of the impressions each interactant holds of the others. As Schlenker (1983) observes, people's social identities can facilitate or impede their social goal achievement in social life.

Given that this is so, people generally recognize that it is to their benefit to monitor and control how they are perceived and regarded by others (Goffman, 1959; Schlenker, 1980; Tedeschi, 1981). Through their self-presentations, they attempt to project images of themselves that they expect will achieve the reactions they desire. People use a variety of modes of conveying impressions of themselves, ranging from what they say about themselves, the attitudes they express, the explanations and attributions they make for their own behavior, their nonverbal expressions and gestures, their appearance, and self-presentational props, such as clothing, home furnishings, and recreational activities. (See Schlenker, 1980, for a detailed discussion of self-presentation.) Nearly every aspect of oneself may be drawn into the service of conveying impressions of oneself to others.

The nature of the impressions an individual attempts to convey depends to a degree upon his or her goals in a particular situation (Schlenker, 1980, 1983). In most instances, people attempt to convey self-images that others will regard as socially desirable. We usually prefer to be seen as friendly, competent, kind, and interested rather than as aloof, incompetent, malicious, and disinterested. In most social settings, socially desirable self-presentations are more likely to elicit the reactions we desire from others present. However, it is sometimes to the individual's advantage to be perceived in what would normally be considered socially *undesirable* ways. For example, a person might wish to be seen as threatening or hostile in order to engender another's compliance (cf. Schelling, 1960) or as incompetent or dependent in order to receive support and protection from others (cf. Braginsky, Braginsky, & Ring, 1969; Schlenker, 1980). The types of impressions that people attempt to convey of themselves depend upon the reactions they desire from others and from the nature of the self-images they believe are most likely to elicit those reactions.

Although nearly all aspects of a person's behavior may reveal information about him or her to others, actions are classified as self-presentational only if the individual *has the goal* of controlling how others perceive him or her (Jones & Pittman, 1982; Schlenker, 1980, 1983). People are not equally motivated to monitor and control how they are regarded by others across all situations. In some social settings, people are relatively unconcerned with conveying particular impressions of themselves, whereas in other encounters their primary goal may be to present particular images of themselves to others. People may have a number of interaction goals in a particular situation—to find out about another interactant, to make a business deal, to reduce loneliness, to seek help, and so on—one of which may be to convey certain impressions of themselves to others.

Schlenker (1980) has stressed that self-presentation does not necessarily imply conscious deception. While it is true that people sometimes attempt to convey self-images that are, from their own standpoint, inaccurate (i.e., that are inconsistent with the way they believe they "really" are), people often engage in self-presentation to assure that others form an *accurate* impression of them. For obvious reasons, people want others to know the best about them. Thus, self-presentation may often involve veridically conveying those aspects of themselves that are expected to elicit the desired reactions from others. Thus, when I want to make a favorable impression upon a woman I know who is fitness-minded, I might casually mention that I run regularly—a perfectly accurate self-presentation, but one that nonetheless is intended to convey a certain impression.

Social Security and Social Anxiety

It may seem to the reader that we have strayed far from our focus on social anxiety. In fact we have not, for the interpersonal processes just described are those from which social insecurities and social anxiety emerge. I have already said that social anxiety results from the prospect or presence of interpersonal evaluation in real or imagined social settings. It should now be clear why people are often apprehensive about others' evaluations of them: How others perceive and evaluate them has important implications for the kinds of social and material outcomes they receive in life. But the prospect or presence of interpersonal evaluation is not *by itself* sufficient to trigger social anxiety. People do not experience social anxiety every time they are under others' explicit or implicit scrutiny. What, then, are the conditions under which social anxiety does and does not occur as a function of interpersonal evaluation?

The self-presentation theory of social anxiety proposes that social anxiety arises whenever

> people are motivated to make a particular impression on others, but doubt that they will do so, having expectations of unsatisfactory impression-relevant reactions from others [Schlenker & Leary, 1982, p. 645; see also, Leary, 1980; Leary & Schlenker, 1981].

This theory locates the immediate cause of social anxiety in the individual's concerns with the kinds of impressions he or she is making and in his or her perceptions of others' reactions to them.

According to this approach, people experience social anxiety when two necessary and sufficient conditions are met. First, the person must be *motivated to make a particular impression on others,* or (in terms we used earlier) must have the *goal* of making a particular impression. As noted above, people do not always have the goal of monitoring and controlling how others perceive them. Not having this goal in a particular social setting, people are not concerned with how they are seen and evaluated by others and, according to the theory, have no chance of experiencing social anxiety in the immediate encounter. Since social anxiety is defined as resulting from the prospect or presence of interpersonal evaluation (see Chapter 1), it can not occur in the absence of evaluative concern. The motivation to make particular impressions on others in the social setting in order to be evaluated and treated in certain ways is the first necessary condition for the experience of social anxiety. All other things being equal, the higher the individual's desire to convey certain impressions, the more likely he or she is to become socially anxious.

Although necessary, the motivation to convey certain impressions of oneself is not sufficient to cause social anxiety. People will not feel socially anxious if they believe they will be successful in conveying the impressions they wish to make and, thus, expect to be regarded in the fashion they desire. There is no interpersonal threat in a situation in which people think they will make the impressions they desire, be evaluated as they wish, and achieve social rewards, no matter how highly motivated they are to manage the impressions they make. Given that the individual has the interpersonal goal of making certain kinds of impressions on others present, they will feel socially anxious only to the degree that they doubt they will successfully do so.

Whenever people have goals, they seek information that will indicate the degree to which they have been successful in achieving the goal. Miller, Galanter, and Pribram (1960) first applied the cybernetic concept of TOTE to goal-directed behavior. TOTE is an acronym for test-operate-test-exit. As organisms engage in goal-directed behaviors, they compare their current state or outcomes against a standard, this comparison constituting the "test" phase of the operation. If the organism's current state or outcomes meet or exceed the standard, the goal has been accomplished and the goal-directed behaviors cease (i.e., the organism "exits" the matching-to-standard process). If, however, the standard is not met, further behavioral operations occur in an attempt to achieve the level of the standard, and the outcome-standard comparison ("test") is made again, and so on. Thus, the comparison of current states with one's standards is an integral part of goal-directed behavior. In the case of self-presentational goals, the goal relevant feedback consists of the real or imagined reactions of others to the individual's self-presentations (Schlenker & Leary, 1982). As they interact, people compare the reactions they perceive they are getting from others to their internal, subjective standards for assessing their interpersonal effectiveness (cf. Bandura, 1977; Carver, 1979).

Perceiving that others' reactions to oneself meet or exceed one's internal standards is tantamount to goal-achievement. The person has made the impressions he or she was motivated to convey, and social anxiety should not occur. (However, since the feedback cues we receive from others may change during the course of an encounter, anxiety may later arise when others' perceived reactions no longer meet our comparison standards.) Only when people believe they are not achieving their self-presentational goals and are not making the impressions they desire will they experience social anxiety. Given that their social and often material outcomes are partially dependent upon the kinds of impressions they create, the perceived failure to make desired impressions will lead people to expect less than satisfactory evaluations and reactions by others.

It should be noted that the individual is seldom able to make an unequivocal judgment of the success of his or her self-presentations in making the desired impressions. Interpersonal feedback is seldom that explicit. As a result, peoples' analyses of their self-presentational efficacy are often based upon expected or purely imagined reactions by others, leaving much room for the personal characteristics of the actor to bias the perception of others' reactions. Put another way, some people are better judges of their interpersonal impact than others. I will return to this important consideration later.

To review, social anxiety is hypothesized to occur when people (a) are motivated to make particular impressions on others, but (b) doubt that they will be successful at doing so. The relationship between these two sets of factors is multiplicative, so that social anxiety will not occur if either factor is zero. Expressed symbolically,

$$SA = f\,[M \times (1 - p)],$$

where

SA = level of social anxiety,
M = level of motivation to make a particular impression, and
p = the subjective probability of making the impressions the individual desires.

IMPLICATIONS

Two implications of the self-presentation approach to social anxiety are noteworthy and underlie the discussion and interpretation of the literature throughout the remainder of this book. First, viewed from a self-presentation perspective, social anxiety is often a reasonable response to certain social settings. Given that other interactants' perceptions have important consequences for people, it makes some degree of sense that they will become apprehensive at the prospect of failing to make particular impressions upon those that they are, for whatever reason, motivated to "impress." The notion that social anxiety may be a reasonable response in some situations runs counter to the theme of much research on the topic. Social anxiety is almost always discussed as if it were indicative of a psychological or social *problem,* or at least that it is somehow irrational or maladaptive to experience apprehension in social encounters. The word "anxiety" itself has connotations of personal weakness and maladjustment. There is nothing inherent in the concept of anxiety in general or social anxiety in particular to warrant such a view. It seems to me quite reasonable to experience anxiety at the prospect of getting an unsatisfactory grade on an important test, losing an election, having a prized possession stolen, or facing any of a host of other unpleasant situations, including potentially aversive *interpersonal* outcomes. The self-presentation approach suggests that social anxiety is a nearly unavoidable byproduct of everyday social life in which people react to one another on the basis of formed impressions. This is not to say that social anxiety is never indicative of socio-psychological difficulties or never causes problems for people. It is simply to note that there is nothing inherently *unreasonable* about social anxiety in many instances.

The second important implication of the self-presentation theory is that all antecedents of social anxiety are hypothesized to produce and exacerbate social anxiety by heightening one or both of the two factors specified in the model. That is, all factors that precipitate feelings of social anxiety do so by increasing the degree to which the person is motivated to make particular impressions upon others and/or heighten their doubts (or, conversely, lower their subjective probability) that they will successfully make those impressions. Any situational or dispositional characteristic that affects one or both of these hypothesized mediators of social anxiety should help determine the individual's level of social anxiety. (Situational factors are characteristics of social settings and the other people in them, such as the sex of other interactants, the novelty of the situation, and the presence of explicit evaluation. Dispositional factors are characteristics, qualities, or attributes of the individual. These may be physical attributes, such as appearance, or psychological attributes, such as intelligence or self-esteem.)

Since this theory posits that the same two sets of factors underlie *all* instances in which people feel socially anxious, we will use the theory as a framework for examining the known causes and correlates of social anxiety. In Chapter 4, we will examine situational and dispositional factors that appear to exacerbate social anxiety by increasing the degree to which people are motivated to convey particular impressions of themselves to others. In Chapter 5, we will turn to the second half of the model and discuss factors that are associated with people's subjective probabilities that they will make the impressions they desire.

4

THE MOTIVATION TO MANAGE IMPRESSIONS

One reason for the current fragmentation of the social anxiety literature is that there has not been an overriding theoretical framework within which to organize and interpret the large amount of information that now exists. Each of the three theoretical perspectives discussed in Chapter 2 was able to handle part of the job, but none was capable of incorporating all empirical findings. Although it is unlikely that *any* theory can truly account for all research findings, it seems that the self-presentation approach introduced in the preceding chapter provides a useful framework for organizing, reviewing, and interpreting the literature. In this chapter, I will use the theory to examine one subset of the known antecedents of social anxiety —those that heighten people's motivation to make particular impressions upon others.

When I say that an individual is "motivated to make a particular impression on others," I mean that he or she has the goal of achieving a desired impression (Schlenker, 1983). As we have already seen, it is with good reason that people are often highly motivated to convey certain impressions of themselves to others. Their self-presentations affect how they are perceived, evaluated, and treated by those with whom they deal. Even so, people do not always have the goal of achieving a particular impression or eliciting a desired response from others. In some social encounters, people seem to care very little if at all about how others regard them. For instance, when people are fully engrossed in an intellectual task, engaged in vigorous physical activity, or directing their attention toward engrossing external events (such as a fire), they are not likely to give much thought to how they are perceived by those who are present. (A brief break in their concentration upon the activity at hand may be accompanied by renewed concern for self-presentation, however.) Likewise, few people are interested in conveying any particular self-image to everybody they meet or even to certain friends and coworkers. Similarly, feelings of anonymity are often accompanied by a lessened concern with others' evaluations (Diener, 1980). In short, many encounters decrease self-presentational concerns.

However, we must be careful not to minimize the degree to which concerns with others' impressions permeate our social lives. Even when people do not appear to be monitoring or controlling how they are being regarded by others (and, thus, might claim that they don't really care how others see them), self-presentational motives are often still present. This can be demonstrated by imagining a situation in which you honestly believe that you have no interest in others' opinions of you. Now picture yourself vomiting in front of all of those people. How would you react? I think most of us would feel greatly embarrassed and would want to leave the situation as quickly as possible. The question is why do people feel so terrible about commiting a social infraction if they don't care in the least about how others regard them? The answer is, of course, that most of us *are* motivated to convey particular impressions of ourselves to others all the time, and the image of a "public vomiter" is not among those we desire to project. In many cases we are not consciously aware of the degree to which we are monitoring and controlling our demeanor until we find ourselves in an embarrassing incident such as this. The fact that one would become embarrassed at all attests to the fact that one would lose face—damage one's public image—in the encounter (Goffman, 1955). The point I want to make is that people are motivated to convey certain, usually desirable impressions of themselves in the majority of their interpersonal dealings whether or not they consciously manage their impressions in all instances.

As Schlenker (1983) notes, the motivation to impress others can vary along a continuum from a total lack of such motivation to an exceptionally high level of motivation. According to the self-presentation approach, the experience of social anxiety is directly related to the extent to which people are motivated to make particular impressions: The more motivated, the more likely they are to feel socially anxious in a particular social setting.

Only one study has experimentally manipulated the degree to which subjects were motivated to make certain impressions upon others in order to examine the effects of this motive upon social anxiety. Prior to having subjects interact over an intercom, Leavy (1980) instructed them either to "act as naturally as possible" (low self-presentational motivation) or to "try to create as favorable an impression on the other subject as you can" (high self-presentational motivation). As predicted by the self-presentation approach to social anxiety, she found that subjects in the high self-presentational motivation condition reported feeling significantly more shy than subjects in the low motivation condition.

In real-life social settings, there are a large number and variety of factors that appear to precipitate or heighten social anxiety by increasing people's motivation to make particular impressions upon others. We will now turn our attention to several such factors.

Focus of Attention: Self-Awareness and Self-Consciousness

Whenever people are awake, they are almost always focusing their attention on something. Right now, you are focusing your attention on the words on this page, although just moments ago you may have been distracted and focusing your attention on something in the room in which you are sitting, on your grumbling stomach, on your watch, or on some other stimulus. Conscious awareness is in continual flux as we shift our attention from one thing to another. In the years since Duval and Wicklund (1972) introduced their theory of self-awareness, a very large literature has emerged that deals with attentional processes and interpersonal behavior. Fortunately, only a portion of the extensive literature concerns us here.

A basic assumption of most theory and research in the area is that it is very difficult if not impossible to focus one's conscious attention on more than one discrete stimulus simultaneously

(Buss, 1980; Duval & Wicklund, 1972). Try to focus your attention on the time of day at *precisely the same moment* that you are thinking about these words. You will be unable to do so, although you may shift your attention back and forth between these stimuli very rapidly.

A second basic assumption has been that objects upon which people may focus their attention may be dichotomized into those that are "external" versus "internal" (e.g., Carver, 1979; Duval & Wicklund, 1972; Fenigstein et al., 1975). On one hand, people may focus their attention upon objects and events that are external to themselves. Another person, an oncoming car, a television show, and the printed pages of a newspaper are examples of things that constitute what we will call an external focus of attention. At other times, people focus their attention upon aspects of themselves, such as their appearance, feelings, thoughts, personality attributes, behavior, and so on, producing a state of self-focused attention (or, often, "objective self-awareness"; Buss, 1980; Duval & Wicklund, 1972; Wicklund, 1975).

Further, it has been argued that, when people direct their attention toward themselves, they may be either privately or publicly self-aware. *Private self-awareness* occurs whenever people attend to aspects of themselves that only they can observe (Buss, 1980). For example, only the experiencing individual can be directly aware of a memory, an idea, a toothache, a taste, personal ethical considerations, a feeling of determination, and so on. Other people may infer what the person is experiencing, but only the individual is able to focus on such stimuli directly. *Public self-awareness* occurs whenever people focus their attention upon aspects of themselves that are easily observed by others. When people think about or observe their own appearance, behavior, mannerisms, speech, and other aspects of their public selves, they are said to be publicly self-aware. For purposes of understanding social anxiety, we will need to focus only on public self-awareness.

PUBLIC SELF-AWARENESS

When people are publicly self-aware, they attend to aspects of themselves that may be observed by others. As a result, they become more conscious of how they might be appearing to others, and thus more concerned with *how others are perceiving and evaluating them* (Buss, 1980; Fenigstein, 1979). Conversely, when an individual is externally focused, he or she is not attending to dimensions of the self and not contemplating others' reactions or the self-relevant implications of them. The individual who is publicly self-focused tends to be highly conscious of how his or her public self is being perceived and evaluated by others and, as a result, is more likely to monitor and control the images they convey in interpersonal encounters. As Fenigstein (1979, p. 75) puts it, "A major consequence of self-consciousness is an increased concern with the presentation of self and the reactions of others to that presentation." As a demonstration of this assertion, Fenigstein (1979) presented female subjects with either favorable or unfavorable feedback about themselves in the context of an interview. The self-awareness of half of the subjects was heightened by exposing them to their own reflections in a mirror—a widely used method of experimentally inducing self-focused attention—whereas the others did not see themselves in the mirror. As expected, subjects reacted more negatively to unfavorable feedback when they had viewed themselves in the mirror than when they had not. There was also a nonsignificant trend for self-focused subjects to respond more positively to favorable feedback. This study supports the notion that, when publicly self-aware, people are more attuned to the interpersonal evaluations of others and react more strongly to them.

By now, the link between public self-awareness and social anxiety should be clear. Given that people are more conscious of how they are being regarded and evaluated when they are publicly self-focused, it follows that public self-awareness would heighten the degree to which people are motivated to convey particular impressions of themselves and thereby increase the likelihood that they will feel socially anxious (Fenigstein, 1979; Leary & Schlenker, 1981; Schlenker & Leary, 1982). In fact, it has been suggested that public self-awareness is a necessary although not sufficient precondition for social anxiety (Buss, 1980; Fenigstein et al., 1975; Leary & Schlenker, 1981). This is true because people will not be motivated to make impressions on others unless they are thinking about the public aspects of themselves and about how others are perceiving and evaluating them. A person who is not currently self-aware is not aware of, thinking about, or concerned with how he or she is being regarded by others (Fenigstein, 1979). In acknowledging this, Buss (1980) argues that the common component of all instances of social anxiety is acute public self-awareness.

The implication of this is that any situational or dispositional factor that leads people to focus attention on their public selves should heighten their motivation to make impressions on those present and increase the chances they will become socially anxious if they doubt that they will do so. Little research has been explicitly conducted on the link between situational inducers of public self-awareness and social anxiety. Nevertheless, a number of hypotheses suggest themselves.

First, the mere realization that others are attending to one's physical appearance or public behavior can quickly induce a state of public self-attention. Indeed, the presence of observers has been used as an experimental manipulation to heighten self-awareness (e.g., Buss, 1980). In everyday life, public self-awareness may occur when others ask about, comment on, or are seen to be observing one's physical features or behavior. The scrutiny of others increases one's desire to act in ways that convey particular impressions.

The impact of others' attention on self-attention and, thus, on social anxiety may help explain why staring usually produces signs of acute discomfort in the target person, often accompanied by an attempt to escape the other's gaze (Ellsworth, Carlsmith, & Henson, 1972; Greenbaum & Rosenfeld, 1978; Strom & Buck, 1979). Aside from the fact that staring is often interpreted as indicative of threat or anger (Ellsworth & Langer, 1976), being the target of a stare causes people to become acutely self-aware. Being under another's intense scrutiny raises self-presentational concerns.

Similarly, simply being the center of attention is usually sufficient to trigger public self-awareness since it attunes the individual to the fact that his or her public self is under observation. It is difficult *not* to think about what others are thinking when one is the center of attention. (How do I look? Is my hair neat? Do I look relaxed? How am I coming across?) Zimbardo (1977) reports that the single situation that people indicate is most likely to make them feel shy is being the center of attention of a large group. In the factor analytic studies of anxiety-inducing situations discussed earlier, "being the center of attention" consistently loads heavily on "social anxiety" factors.

Presumably, such situations are highly anxiety-arousing for at least two reasons. First, being the center of attention induces public self-awareness, increasing the actor's desire to make appropriate impressions. On top of that, many if not most people tend to doubt their ability to handle such situations adroitly. The demands of being the center of attention are somewhat different than those encountered in more common face-to-face interactions. As a result, many people may expect to project a less-than-satisfactory image of themselves and receive less-than-optimal evaluative reactions from those who are observing them. Being the center of attention delivers a "double whammy" that sends social anxiety soaring in many people.

Public self-awareness is also particularly high when people believe they possess a physical or social stigma that draws others' attention to them (Buss, 1980). A physical stigma is an easily observed physical defect. A stigma may include major and relatively permanent defects, such as severe handicaps, missing limbs, or facial deformities, or relatively minor and, often, transitory "defects" such as black eyes, blemishes, a few extra pounds, or a new hairstyle that didn't quite work. A person who possesses (or at least believes he or she possesses) a physical stigma is likely to be publicly self-aware much of the time. A social stigma refers to "defects" in a person's social identity—negative information about the person that is known by others. Having to face someone who just learned that you are illegitimate, performed numerous unfortunate actions while quite inebriated, abused your children, were fired for incompetence, and so on is to feel stigmatized.

Because the stigmatized person is highly self-aware, he or she is sensitive to others' real or imagined evaluations, highly motivated to make as good an impression as possible, and likely to feel socially anxious. (Of course, over time, people with a permanent stigma may feel less self-conscious about it.) Not only does possession of a physical or social stigma induce public self-awareness, it also makes people doubt that others will evaluate them favorably and thereby creates both of the conditions needed for social anxiety. When viewed in this manner, the anxiety experienced by the adolescent who discovers that he or she has sprouted huge pimples just before the senior prom is a predictable manifestation of social anxiety. The adolescent is highly motivated to make a particular impression, but believes that the pimples will make him or her unable to do so. The impact of physical and social stigmata upon affect and behavior is a ripe topic for future research.

Many stimuli present in social settings cause public self-awareness in most people. Consider how quickly people's attention shifts to themselves when a camera (particularly a movie camera) is pointed in their direction. It is very difficult for most people to concentrate on whatever they are saying or doing once they realize that their public selves are being photographed, filmed, or videotaped. While desperately trying to appear natural, people adjust their hair, straighten their clothes, attempt to appear pleasant, become acutely aware of their posture, gestures, and expression, and otherwise work hard to appear photogenic. Similarly, the presence of a microphone makes people aware of their speech—its tone, pattern, pace, use of "ahs" and "uhs," word usage, and so on. Since people don't normally focus closely on their speech as they talk, conscious attention to one's own voice can be quite unnerving and disruptive.

Mirrors and other reflective surfaces also make people highly self-aware (see Buss, 1980, for a review). When passing a reflective store window, for example, people tend to quickly inspect their appearance and make whatever adjustments in their clothing, posture, or hair are deemed necessary; only moments earlier, they were totally nonconscious of the public aspects of themselves.

Interacting with others in the presence of reflective surfaces provides a constant reminder of oneself as a social object that is being seen and evaluated by others. I remember having to speak to a psychology class on my very first job interview in a classroom that had a large mirror across the rear wall. Although I was adequately prepared for my lecture and felt reasonably confident about my ability to deliver it well, I faltered upon reaching the lectern and being confronted with my full-length reflection in the mirror. The experience of public self-awareness was quite intense. Not only was I the center of the class' attention and under the scrutiny of members of the psychology faculty who were interviewing me, but I was faced with my own image throughout the talk. The combination of these factors increased my self-presentational concerns and, thus, my level of social anxiety. Each time I glanced at my reflection, I found myself scrutinizing my appearance and behavior and wondering how I was being perceived and evaluated by my audience. Luckily, since I was lecturing about social anxiety, I was able to use my own discomfort as an example of the effect of public self-awareness on feelings of social anxiety.

PUBLIC SELF-CONSCIOUSNESS

While the state of public self-awareness may be induced by a number of stimuli in the social setting and heightened by the presence of stigma, individuals differ in the degree to which such factors actually trigger self-awareness. Consistent with Buss's (1980) use of the terms, we will use public *self-awareness* to refer to the *state* of focusing one's attention upon public aspects of the self, and use the term public *self-consciousness* to refer to individual differences in the *tendency* to be publicly self-aware across situations and time.

The trait of public self-consciousness is typically measured by the "public" subscale of the Self-Consciousness Scale (Fenigstein et al., 1975). This scale is a seven-item measure of the degree to which people tend to think about public aspects of themselves and contemplate others' reactions to them. Questions include items such as "I'm concerned about what other people think of me," "I'm usually aware of my appearance," and "One of the last things I do before I leave my house is look in the mirror." The public self-consciousness scale is highly reliable (Fenigstein et al., 1975), demonstrates strong evidence of construct and criterion validity (see Carver & Glass, 1976), and has been used in studies of a number of social psychological phenomena.

People who score high in public self-consciousness think more about public aspects of themselves, are more attuned to others' evaluations of them, and are more concerned with managing their impressions than people who score low on the scale (Buss, 1980; Fenigstein, 1979; Fenigstein et al., 1975; Leavy, 1980). For example, Fenigstein (1979) found that high publicly self-conscious females were more strongly affected by being shunned by other individuals than were low self-conscious females. Miller and Cox (1982) showed that women who scored high in public self-consciousness were more likely to use makeup than less publicly self-conscious women. Since makeup is used in the service of improving one's appearance, it makes sense that people who are more cognizant of others' reactions to their public appearance would try harder to improve their social images. Similarly, high public self-consciousness is also associated with the emphasis one places on clothing (Solomon & Schopler, 1982).

Viewed from the perspective of the self-presentation theory of social anxiety, publicly self-conscious people are generally more highly motivated to make particular impressions upon others (Leary & Schlenker, 1981; Leavy, 1980). Thus, it should not be surprising to find that public self-consciousness is associated with higher levels of social anxiety. Indeed, several studies report a significant correlation between scores on the public Self-Consciousness Scale and measures of dispositional social anxiousness, including the social anxiety subscale of the Self-Consciousness Scale (Buss, 1980; Fenigstein, 1979; Fenigstein et al., 1975; Pilkonis, 1977a; Turner, 1977), the Interaction Anxiousness and Audience Anxiousness Scales (Leary, 1983a), the Shyness Scale (Cheek & Buss, 1981), the Social Reticence Scale (Jones &

Russell, 1982), and a one-item measure of self-reported shyness (Pilkonis, 1977a).[1] As Fenigstein et al. (1975) suggest, public self-consciousness may be necessary for an individual to experience social anxiety. This is because some awareness of others' potential reactions to oneself is necessary in order for the individual to have the goal of making impressions upon others.

SELF-FOCUS AND INTERPERSONAL BEHAVIOR

To the degree that a person is focused on him- or herself, attention is directed *away* from external events. Being distracted from the stimuli in a particular social setting may impair one's ability to respond appropriately to social contingencies. The socially anxious person may often be so preoccupied with him- or herself that he or she does not direct sufficient attention toward what others are saying and doing. If a parallel may be drawn between social anxiety and test anxiety, it has been shown that self-deprecating thoughts detract from the anxious test-taker's ability to devote full attention to the test itself, thus debilitating performance (e.g., Mandler & Watson, 1966; Wine, 1971).

In a study that examined the attention of socially anxious individuals, Hatvany, Souza e Silva, & Zimbardo (1981) had shy males (identified by the single self-report item on the Stanford Shyness Survey) listen to a speech under one of three evaluative conditions. Some subjects believed that the female speaker was being evaluated, others thought they themselves were being evaluated, and the remaining third were unsure regarding who was being evaluated. Compared to subjects identified as "nonshy," the "shy" subjects recalled significantly less of the content of the woman's speech, but only when they believed that *they* themselves were the target of evaluation in the experiment. Apparently, a high state of self-attention and preoccupation prevented shy subjects who thought they were under scrutiny from devoting full attention to the speech.

This finding suggests interesting implications for education. To the degree that anxious preoccupation interferes with cognitive processing (see Weinstein, Cubberly, & Richardson, 1982), social-evaluative concerns may impair learning. Thus, in a class in which the teacher routinely calls on students to speak or answer questions, socially anxious students may be so worried about being called on that they have difficulty attending to the material being discussed. In addition, once they are asked to speak, their self-preoccupation and apprehension may hamper their ability to formulate a cogent response.

As we will explore in greater detail in later chapters, the literature on public self-awareness, self-consciousness and social anxiety suggests that it may be possible to reduce high social anxiousness by helping people focus their attention *away* from themselves. Although it can be argued that a certain level of awareness of how one is coming across to others is necessary for smooth and effective interactions, it is often neither necessary nor desirable. People who are unable to enjoy a lively party because they are constantly wondering about how they are coming across to others are inappropriately self-aware. It may be possible to help highly self-conscious individuals learn to focus their attention less on themselves and more upon others in social encounters, thereby reducing the likelihood that they will experience social anxiety.

Value of Hoped-For Outcomes

When people have the goal of projecting certain images of themselves to others, it is usually because they expect that the kinds of impressions they make will affect how others evaluate and treat them. People monitor and control their self-presentations in order to maximize their social rewards while minimizing their social costs (Schlenker, 1980). It follows that the degree to which people are motivated to convey particular impressions of themselves to others will be affected by the perceived *value* of the outcomes they desire to receive. The more valuable or important others' evaluations and reactions are to the individual, the more concerned the person should be with obtaining those outcomes, and the more motivated the person should be to convey impressions that they expect will produce them.

At one extreme are situations in which people believe that they have nothing whatsoever to gain or lose as the result of a particular social encounter. Others' perceptions, evaluations, and treatment of them are of absolutely no concern. In such situations, people should not be motivated to convey any particular impressions of themselves and, according to the self-presentation theory, should not experience social anxiety.

At the other extreme are encounters in which the social and/or economic stakes are very high. In such situations, the consequences of projecting "appropriate" self-images to those who are in the position to reward and punish are substantial. When the value of hoped-for outcomes is very high, individuals are strongly motivated to come across in certain ways and, thus, have a high likelihood of feeling socially anxious. Under these circumstances, people are likely to react to even minor flubs with discomfort and nervousness whereas they would not give them a second thought under other circumstances.

All other things being equal, people are more highly motivated to manage their impressions when they believe that how they are perceived by others has important consequences for them. As a result, people should be more likely to experience social anxiety and experience it more intensely as the potential positive and negative outcomes they may receive from others in the encounter become greater. Nearly all of the other factors discussed in this chapter can be regarded as affecting social anxiety by increasing the value or importance of the outcomes people desire to obtain as a result of their participation in interpersonal encounters.

Initial Encounters

Most people are convinced of the importance of first impressions, as exemplified by adages such as "Put your best foot forward" and "You never get a second chance to make a first impression." Research shows that the layperson's intuitions are correct: Information about a person that is received first is weighed more heavily in forming an impression of the individual than information that is received later (Jones & Goethals, 1972). According to one view (Asch, 1946), once people have obtained initial information and begin to form an impression of someone, they tend to interpret information received later in a manner consistent with the initial impression. For example, if you initially form an impression of a woman as kind and witty, you are likely to interpret her mildly sarcastic remarks as harmless jests. However, if your initial impression is that she is cold and cutting, you may interpret those same mildly sarcastic comments as cruel jokes made at another's expense. Your initial impression provided a context in which later behavior was interpreted. In addition, first impressions carry inordinate weight because observers tend to discount or "tune out" information about others that is inconsistent with what they already believe about them (Anderson, 1965). Once people have formed an initial impression of someone, they place less emphasis on later information that does not jibe with their first impression.

As can be seen, the emphasis that most people put on making a good first impression is not misplaced; the primacy effect in person perception warrants attention to the kinds of impressions others form during initial encounters. Unfortunately, one consequence of recognizing the importance of making good first impressions is that people are highly motivated to manage their impressions when they meet others for the first time, resulting in an increased likelihood of social anxiety. Research findings attest that meeting people for the first time, being introduced to new people, and interacting with strangers are highly anxiety-arousing situations for many people (e.g., Curran, 1977; Jones & Russell, 1982; Strahan, 1974; Zimbardo, 1977).

Characteristics of Other Interactants

Social psychological research has consistently demonstrated that people's social responses are strongly affected by the perceived characteristics of other interactants. In the course of interpersonal encounters, people respond not only to what other interactants say and do, but also to their personal characteristics, such as their race, sex, status, height, and so on. In the case of social anxiety, people often report feeling more anxious when dealing with authorities, members of the other sex, experts, physically attractive people, and those of high status (Zimbardo, 1977). Why are some people perceived as more threatening in social situations than others? There are two general reasons which correspond to the two factors in the self-presentation theory of social anxiety: People are often more highly motivated to make particular impressions upon those who possess characteristics such as those listed above, but furthermore people are more likely to doubt that they can make desired impressions upon such individuals. I will discuss the first reason in this section, but leave the second until Chapter 5.

People seem to value the opinions, evaluations, and reactions of certain kinds of people more highly than they do those of others. For example, most people are more concerned with how they are perceived, evaluated, and treated by those whom they regard as attractive, competent, socially desirable, and powerful than by those with less desirable characteristics. The evaluations of significant others are often perceived as more diagnostic and valid than the reactions of undesirable others. Whose evaluation would a person take more seriously—that of a talented, competent, and socially desirable individual, or that of an incompetent, inept, socially undesirable one? Clearly, people place more importance on the evaluations of socially desirable others. Since others' evaluations have effects upon a person's own self-esteem and feelings of worth, they would be more motivated to obtain positive evaluative reactions and avoid negative evaluative reactions from desirable than from undesirable others, all other things being equal. As a result, they should be more motivated to convey particular impressions of themselves and more likely to feel socially anxious when dealing with competent, high status, and attractive people. Put simply, it is worth more to be liked by desirable than undesirable people.

Another reason why people are more likely to value the evaluative reactions of competent, powerful, high-status others is that such individuals are often in the position to mediate valuable rewards and punishments. Employers, teachers, supervisors, and others in positions of authority are likely to bestow positive outcomes upon those who suitably impress them and negative outcomes upon those who do not. Thus, it is not surprising that people are often concerned about how they are being perceived and evaluated by authority figures.

Perhaps the personal characteristic that most commonly precipitates or exacerbates social anxiety in our culture is the sex of the other interactant. A high proportion of the American population reports that they are often uncomfortable interacting socially with those of the other sex. In a group of nearly 4000 randomly sampled undergraduates, Arkowitz et al. (1978) found that 37% of the men and 25% of the women indicated that they were "somewhat" or "very" anxious about dating, and approximately 50% of each sex said they would be interested in attending a program designed to increase their comfort in dating situations. Nearly half of another sample rated cross-sex interactions as "high" in social difficulty (Glass et al., 1976), and 64% of Zimbardo's (1977) shy respondents indicated that people of the other sex caused them to feel shy. Given the prevalence of such concerns, it is not surprising that a large literature has arisen around the topic of *heterosocial anxiety* (or, often, heterosexual-social anxiety) which is defined as anxiety arising from real, anticipated, or imagined interactions with those of the other sex (Leary & Dobbins, 1983).

Viewed from the self-presentation perspective, it is easy to see why cross-sex encounters are highly anxiety-arousing. In a society that places a strong emphasis on male-female relationships, sex appeal, and heterosexuality, those of the opposite sex are in the position to mediate valued social rewards. When people make the "appropriate" impressions upon those of the other sex, they are likely to receive self-affirming feedback indicating that they are socially and/or sexually desirable—feedback that is highly valued in our culture. In addition, success in one's heterosocial dealings demonstrates one's social worth to onlookers; in some circles, a major benefit of attracting members of the opposite sex is to impress one's own friends. And, of course, being perceived in favorable ways by the other sex has the potential to result in acquisition of a dating, romantic, sexual, or marital partner, along with the attendant benefits of such a relationship. The emphasis that much of Western culture places on female-male relations leads people to be highly motivated to make particular impressions upon those of the other sex.

Although the importance of heterosocial rewards and punishments accounts for many instances in which people control their self-presentations for those of the other sex, it is curious that men and women often appear to be highly concerned with their social images in heterosocial encounters even when there is no possibility of receiving social rewards or punishments. (This is true of other kinds of encounters, but we will, for the moment, restrict our discussion to heterosocial situations.) Watch people on the beach suck in their stomachs as they walk by attractive members of the other sex, even though they may have no intention of actually interacting with them. Similarly, people sometimes seem interested in conveying certain self-images to perfect strangers in the grocery store, on airplanes, and on the street. They are clearly motivated to make certain impressions, but why?

Even when people are not directly affected by others' evaluations of them, they are able to *imagine* the kinds of impressions others are forming. And, although it seems irrational, people are sometimes as distressed about these imagined reactions as they are about actual ones, even when there are no material or social outcomes at stake. There are at least two ways of interpreting this observation. First, since others' evaluations of the individual are often associated with real positive or negative consequences for him or her, others' real or imagined evaluations acquire what behaviorists call secondary reinforcing and punishing properties. (A secondary or conditioned reinforcer is one that acquires its reinforcing qualities by having been associated with other reinforcers.) Thus, we take pride when others view our accomplishments and feel ashamed when others learn of our transgressions even though we may receive absolutely no direct or indirect feedback from them.

Second, a central assumption of symbolic interactionism—from which the self-presentation approach springs—is that people's views of themselves are strongly affected by how they believe they are perceived and evaluated by others (Cooley, 1922). Thus, others' real or imagined perceptions and evaluations have implications for one's own self-concept and self-esteem. If we assume that people generally desire to enhance and maintain their self-esteem (Wells & Marwell, 1976), it follows that they will be motivated to behave in ways that will result in real or imagined positive reactions from others. It deflates one's self-esteem to even *imagine* that one is not being viewed in desired ways. Thus, when walking down the beach, I suck in my stomach to avoid the imagined negative evaluations of women who are watching me. It is more rewarding for me to imagine that other people think I look reasonably attractive than to believe they view me as a disgusting slob.

Salience of Evaluation

Social settings differ in the degree to which interpersonal evaluation is salient. In some encounters, evaluation is present but implicit, as when it is obvious to people that others are "sizing them up" for one reason or another. (I am reminded here of instances in which I met a date's parents for the first time.) In other settings the evaluation is explicit, such as when a person is being interviewed for a job or is participating in a public speaking contest. In such situations, everyone present, including the target of the evaluation, knows that an evaluation is occurring. In yet other cases, it appears that interactants are not evaluating one another at all.

Whether implicit or explicit, evaluative overtones should increase the target's desire to project certain self-images to the evaluators compared to encounters that are not obviously evaluative. Since evaluation by others carries the potential for positive and negative outcomes for the individual, people should be highly concerned with the impressions others are forming and, thus, be more likely to feel socially anxious.

Although no research has directly addressed this notion, examples are readily available. A man who is normally quite comfortable chatting with his boss might suddenly find himself unusually anxious and awkward interacting with the boss shortly before promotions and raises are to be awarded. The immediacy of the supervisor's evaluation creates a greater desire to make the appropriate impressions. Similarly, a woman may normally feel at ease when speaking before large groups, but find herself experiencing intense audience anxiety while giving a campaign speech shortly before an election in which she is a candidate. (Are presidential candidates more socially anxious during the nationwide televised debates than they are in other, less crucial campaign appearances? The present model would suggest this hypothesis. Inasmuch as social anxiety arises from the prospect or presence of interpersonal evaluation, situational cues that increase the salience of the evaluation should increase the likelihood that the actor will experience social anxiety.

Centrality of Impressions to Self-Concept

People's self-concepts consist of a number of self-constructs or self-schema. These are the categories people use to classify and organize information about themselves. For example, a woman's self-concept might include the constructs "hard-working, generous, athletic, and impatient." These self-schemas are generalizations based upon observed regularities in her behavior. Instead of recalling each and every little fact about themselves, people use a limited number of self-constructs to identify what they are like.

The constructs people hold of themselves may be arranged in a hierarchy according to how important or central the constructs are to the person's sense of identity. Put another way, some self-constructs are more important to an individual than are others. For example, the construct that one is an "animal-lover" may be more important to one's sense of self than the construct that one is relatively "athletic." Although both constructs may be equally descriptive, the individual values one attribute more than the other and considers it more important to his or her self-concept. Although there is not yet any empirical evidence to bear upon this hypothesis, it seems likely that people are more highly motivated to convey impressions of themselves that are more (rather than less) central to their self-concepts. Using the example above, a person might be more interested in being perceived by others as an animal-lover than as an athlete.

Creating the desired impressions (of being an animal-lover, for example) would allow them to receive the satisfaction of being regarded by others in ways that they themselves consider personally important. In addition, successfully projecting a social identity that embodies constructs central to one's self-concept provides the individual with self-validating feedback. It is important for people to receive confirmation that they are the things they believe and desire themselves to be. One source of such confirmation is others' reactions to one's self-presentations. If other people accept at face value the images people project, external validation for one's self-constructs has been obtained. Thus, people will be motivated to project images of themselves that will result in the confirmation of important self-constructs from others. If the self-construct "animal-lover" is central to a woman's self-concept, she may wish to convey to others the image of a person who likes animals. When other people comment, "It sure seems you like animals" or "It's great that you give so much time to the humane society," she receives feedback indicating that others regard her as an animal-lover as well. Such feedback regarding attributes that are central to one's self-concept is quite rewarding—more so than feedback regarding constructs that are peripheral to one's sense of identity.

Number of Others Present

All other things being equal, people are more likely to report feeling socially anxious as the number of other people present increases. People generally indicate that they are more anxious at large parties than at small parties, and when speaking or performing before large than small audiences (Knight & Borden, 1978;

Latane & Harkins, 1976; Zimbardo, 1977). Although social anxiety increases with the number of interactants, the impact of each additional person added to the situation might be expected to have less and less of an effect upon the individual's level of anxiety. A person who is at a party with 25 other people might be more likely to feel nervous than if he or she were at a party with 5 others. However, the addition of those 20 additional partiers would have minimal, if any impact upon the individual's anxiety if there were already 200 people at the party. Similarly, giving a speech in front of 20 people may be more anxiety-producing than speaking for a group of 10, but the addition of those 10 to an audience of 800 is not likely to have any discernible effect upon the speaker.

Research by Latane and his colleagues (see Latane, 1981, for a review) clearly demonstrates this effect. Within a number of quite disparate social contexts (e.g., conformity, prosocial behavior, crowding in rats, tipping in restaurants), constant increases in the number of others present have less and less social impact upon the individual's responses. Latane compares this effect to the principle of marginally decreasing utility in economics: A given amount of money is worth less the more money one already has.

In one study by Latane and Harkins (1976), college students were asked to imagine that they were to recite a memorized poem in front of an audience of either 1, 2, 4, 8, or 16 people. They were to indicate how nervous they would feel reciting the poem by adjusting the brightness of a light or the loudness of a tone. (This procedure, called cross-modality matching, was adapted from psychophysical research.) Results showed that estimated social tension (i.e., anxiety) was greater before imagined larger audiences, but that there was a marginally decreasing effect of audience size. In other words, although subjects indicated that they would feel about twice as tense in front of 4 than 2 people, they were only about three times as tense in front of 8 than 2, and only about four times as tense when reciting in front of 16 as 2. (Another way to say this is that tension appeared to increase in proportion to the square root of the number of people in the audience.)

An early study of stuttering by Porter (1939) showed that speech disfluencies—presumably indicative of subjective anxiety—increased with audience size. Reanalyzing Porter's data, Latane (1981) found that, like subjective tension, the stuttering of Porter's subjects fit a deaccelerating curve. Stuttering increased in proportion to the cube root of audience size.

Research by Knight and Borden (1978) suggests that audience size interacts with audience expertise in heightening social anxiety. They had undergraduates sing "Row, Row, Row Your Boat" in front of audiences of 1, 3, or 8 other students. In addition, subjects were told that their audience consisted of students who were either high or low in musical ability. Analyses of subjects' self-ratings of anxiety showed main effects of audience size and audience expertise, which were qualified by an audience size by expertise interaction. Audience size had a significant effect upon anxiety ratings only when the audience was believed to be high in musical ability. Subjects singing in front of a high ability audience were more anxious when there were 8 rather than 1 or 3 people watching them. No differences in anxiety ratings were obtained as a function of audience size when subjects believed the audience was low in ability. An effect might have been found with larger audiences; presumably, most people would feel more socially anxious when singing for 100 than 3 people, no matter what the audience's level of musical ability.

Although no researchers have yet asked specifically *why* increases in audience size result in heightened social anxiety, the self-presentation approach suggests two possibilities. First, it seems likely that larger groups increase people's motivation to make desired impressions upon those present. The interpersonal evaluations of many people have the potential for greater impact upon the individual than the evaluations of just a few. Put another way, it is better to make a good impression, but worse to make a bad impression, upon 50 as opposed to 5 other people, for example. Thus, we would expect to find that people are more highly motivated to manage their impressions as the number of observers increases, all other things being equal. Further, Latane's (1981) theory of social impact would lead us to expect that the relationship between audience size and the motivation to make impressions upon those present is a marginally decreasing one, similar to the relationship he identified between audience size and anxiety (Latane & Harkins, 1976).

A second reason why social anxiety increases with audience size might be that most people are less confident of their ability to project desired images of themselves as the size of the group increases. Speaking to larger groups whether in public speaking or semiconversational settings such as parties often requires the individual to be a bit of a storyteller or performer. The interpersonal skills required in such settings are somewhat different than those needed for more common contingent conversations. As a result, individuals who are comfortable conversing with a handful of others may experience acute anxiety when they become the focus of attention of a large group and are forced to "perform" (i.e., tell a story, anecdote, or joke to an "audience") rather than merely converse. Relatively few individuals have had the experience needed to hone their public speaking skills.

Needs for Social Approval

The kind of impression an individual is motivated to convey to others depends largely upon his or her goals in the encounter and the reward-punishment contingencies of the situation. In some instances, people will be motivated to try to project social images that others will regard as socially desirable, whereas in others, they will want to appear undesirable in order to achieve their interaction goals. Instances of the first type are undoubtedly more common than those of the second. People are usually more motivated to obtain others' approval, acceptance, and affection than others' disapproval and rejection. In addition, certain characteristics of social settings and of people's personalities appear to heighten the degree to which they are motivated to seek others' approval and/or avoid their disapproval. Since people will manage their impressions to a greater degree when their need for approval is high (Schlenker, 1980), factors that heighten people's motivation to seek approval should be associated with increased social anxiety.

SITUATIONAL FACTORS

Sometimes people seem not to care about others' evaluations of them whereas at other times they seem starved for affection and acceptance. There is evidence, for example, that recent failure experiences heighten people's attempts to gain approval from others. Schneider (1969) showed that subjects who believed they had failed a test of social sensitivity described themselves more positively to an interviewer (who did not know their scores, but was later to reevaluate them) than subjects who believed they performed well on the test. In addition, subjects who thought they had failed the test presented themselves more positively to the interviewer when they believed that the interviewer would give them feedback about his evaluation than when they thought he would not. Apparently, subjects who failed wanted an indication of approval from the interviewer and managed their impressions in ways designed to attain it.

A study by Baumeister and Jones (1978) also examined how people manage their impressions following failure. People who publicly fail at a task are in a self-presentational quandary. They are highly motivated to make particular impressions upon others (in order to attain their approval), but their self-presentations are constrained by what the others know about their failure. They cannot hope to convince others that they should be evaluated highly on attributes implicated in the failure; their self-aggrandizing claims would be disregarded. Baumeister and Jones found that people in such a situation strike a happy balance. While projecting accurate (i.e., negative) information about themselves on attributes related to their failure, people enhance their self-presentations on personal attributes not related to their failure. Such a self-presentational strategy allows people to compensate for publicly known unfavorable information about them. This finding again demonstrates that people are motivated to seek others' approval after failure and will manage their impressions to do so as best they can under the circumstances.

There are at least two major reasons why failure heightens the desire for social approval. First, if one's shortcomings are public knowledge, the individual will want to enhance his or her image in others' eyes in order to repair the damage to social identity caused by the failure. Since others' evaluations can have important consequences for the individual, people are highly motivated to forestall negative social repercussions of failure by improving their tarnished image (Goffman, 1955).

Second, people's feelings of *self-worth* are partially dependent upon others' evaluations of them (Cooley, 1922; Coopersmith, 1967; Mead, 1934). Others' appraisals are a major determinant of how people perceive and evaluate themselves (Backman, Secord, & Pierce, 1963; Haas & Maehr, 1965; Videbeck, 1960). Since people's feelings about themselves are partially based upon how they believe they are regarded by others, people can raise their self-esteem by obtaining positive evaluations from others. Following a failure in which one's self-perceptions of competence, control, and worth are called into question, successfully obtaining favorable reactions from others may lead the individual to feel better about him- or herself. As a result, after having failed people are often motivated to make particular impressions that will elicit others' acceptance and approval.

Since people are more highly desirous of obtaining others' approval after they have failed in some way, we might expect them to be more susceptible to feelings to social anxiety. Not only are they highly motivated to convey particular impressions, but the failure itself may lead them to doubt that they will be successful at making the impressions they desire. This hypothesis warrants future attention.

DISPOSITIONAL FACTORS

Although the degree to which people desire approval from others fluctuates over situations and time, some people are characteristically more interested in obtaining social approval and/or avoiding disapproval than are other people (Berger, Levin, Jacobsen, & Milham, 1977; Crowne & Marlowe, 1964). Since people who are high in need for approval (as measured by the Social Desirability Scale, for example; Crowne & Marlowe, 1964) are more motivated to make good impressions upon others, they should be more likely to experience social anxiety than people low in need for approval. In addition, people who are high in need for approval possess other characteristics that may predispose them to become socially anxious more frequently than lows. High need for approval individuals tend to lack the "confidence, assertiveness, and skill to make the best out of social situations" (Schlenker, 1980, p. 79). They also tend to be defensive, are not regarded as friendly by others, and often lack certain expressive skills as well (Crowne & Marlowe, 1964; Zaidel & Mehrabian, 1969). Coupled with a high degree of concern about the impressions they make on others, these characteristics may render high need for approval individuals highly prone to feelings of social anxiety.

Unfortunately, there is a problem involved in testing this hypothesis. Since people who are high in need for approval want to appear in socially desirable ways, they may be reluctant to admit that they are highly socially anxious. As a result, high need for approval people may misrepresent themselves on self-report measures that, if answered veridically, would portray them in a negative light. (Indeed, the Social Desirability Scale measures need for approval by examining the degree to which people endorse highly desirable self-statements that are almost certain to be false, such as "No matter who I'm talking to, I'm always a good listener.") Consistent with this possibility is the finding that need for approval is *negatively* correlated with shyness ($r = -.27$, $p < .05$; Jones & Russell, 1982).

Nevertheless, we have already seen that people who are excessively (i.e., "irrationally") concerned about being accepted and approved of by others tend to be higher in social anxiousness than those who are lower in their need for acceptance (e.g., Ellis, 1962; Goldfried & Sobocinski, 1975). Thus, our earlier discussion of the role of irrational beliefs in social anxiety is applicable here (see Chapter 2). The self-presentation theory easily subsumes the "irrational belief" version of the cognitive approach to social anxiety. In brief, high needs for acceptance and approval are associated with social anxiety because such needs motivate the individual to attempt to project particular impressions to others.

Fear of Negative Evaluation

A construct closely related to need for approval is fear of negative evaluation. People differ in the degree to which they become apprehensive at the prospect of receiving negative evaluations from others. Some people are often worried about how others perceive and evaluate them, whereas others seldom give other people's views of them a second thought. Since people who are highly apprehensive about being evaluated negatively are more concerned with making good impressions on others and try harder to do so (Leary, 1980), one would expect a strong relationship between measures of evaluation apprehension and social anxiety.

Data from a number of sources support this hypothesized relationship. In a study of highly socially anxious individuals, Nichols (1974) observed that the most common characteristic of these subjects was sensitivity to and fearfulness of receiving disapproval and criticism from others. Similarly, Goldfried and Sobocinski (1975) found moderate correlations between subjects' endorsement of the "irrational" belief that it is essential to be loved and approved of by others (presumably indicative of a concern for others' evaluations) and scores on the Social Avoidance and Distress Scale ($r = .36$, $p < .01$) and the Personal Report of Confidence as a Speaker ($r = .33$, $p < .01$).

Watson and Friend (1969) constructed the Fear of Negative Evaluation (FNE) Scale to assess the degree to which people experience apprehension at the prospect of receiving negative evaluations from others. (A brief version of the FNE Scale can be found in Leary, 1983d.) High FNE people tend to endorse items such as "I am frequently afraid that others will notice my shortcomings" and "I am afraid others will not approve of me," whereas low FNE's tend to indicate that "I rarely worry about seeming foolish to others." Research has shown that scores on the FNE are strongly related to the motivation to seek approval and avoid disapproval from others. Compared to subjects classified as low FNE, high FNE individuals worked harder on a boring letter-substitution task when they believed that hard work would be explicitly approved by their group leader (Watson & Friend, 1969); attempted to avoid potentially self-threatening social comparison information to a greater degree (Friend & Gilbert, 1973); indicated they feel worse about being evaluated negatively (Smith & Sarason, 1975), prefer to be in a positive asymmetrical relationship—being liked by another more than one likes the other—rather than a balanced relationship (Smith & Campbell, 1973), and are more concerned with making good impressions on others (Leary, 1980). Also, FNE scores correlate $+.77$ ($p<.01$) with social approval-seeking as measured by Jackson's Personality Research Form (Watson & Friend, 1969). Taken together, these findings portray the high FNE individual as one who is highly motivated both to gain approval and to avoid disapproval (Watson & Friend, 1969). Thus, it would be expected that FNE would be associated with both situational and dispositional social anxiety.

Scores on the FNE correlate moderately to highly with several measures of social anxiousness, including the Social Avoidance and Distress Scale (Leary, 1980; Montgomery & Haemmerlie, 1982; Watson & Friend, 1969), the social anxiety subscale of the Self-Consciousness Scale (Leavy, 1980), the Interaction Anxiousness Scale (Leary, 1983a), and measures of audience anxiousness (Goldfried & Sobocinski, 1975; Leary, 1983a).[2] These correlations clearly implicate fear of negative evaluation as an important factor in social anxiety.

In an experimental study, Leary (1980) had high and low FNE subjects interact with another naive subject under conditions in which either the way to act in order to make a good impression upon the other subject was made explicit or was left ambiguous. An FNE measurement (high-low) by ambiguity (high-low) interaction on self-reported relaxation during the conversation showed that whereas low FNE subjects reported being equally relaxed whether they knew what kind of image to project or not, high FNE subjects felt significantly less relaxed when they did not know how to act in order to make a good impression on the other subject than when they did know how to respond. People who are high in fear of negative evaluation appear to become more anxious when they do not know how to make good impressions on others.

Summary

The self-presentation theory of social anxiety posits that one necessary condition for the experience of social anxiety is that the individual be motivated to make particular impressions on others. Any situational or dispositional variable that heightens the motivation to impression manage should increase the likelihood that the person will become anxious. Several such factors were considered in this chapter, including public self-awareness and self-consciousness, the value of the outcomes the individual hopes to attain through interactions with others, initial encounters, the personal characteristics of other interactants, the salience of evaluative overtones in a particular encounter, the centrality of the projected image to the actor's self-concept, the number of other people who are present, situational and dispositional antecedents of the need for social approval, and the degree to which the individual is apprehensive about being evaluated negatively by other people. In each instance, we saw that the factors that lead people to want to convey particular impressions of themselves are precisely those factors that precipitate and exacerbate social anxiety, thus lending support to the self-presentation approach.

Notes

1. Correlations between scores on the Public Self-Consciousness Scale and measures of social anxiousness and shyness range from .18 to .37, p's$<.05$.
2. Correlations between scores on the Fear of Negative Evaluation Scale and measures of social anxiousness and shyness range from .28 to .77, p's$<.05$.

5

SELF-PRESENTATIONAL EFFICACY

To repeat the central proposition of the self-presentation theory of social anxiety: Social anxiety arises in real or imagined social settings when people are motivated to make a particular impression on others but doubt that they will do so, having expectations of unsatisfactory impression-relevant reactions from others (Schlenker & Leary, 1982). As this proposition notes, just being highly motivated to make particular impressions on others is not in itself sufficient to trigger social anxiety. I may be extremely interested in another person regarding me in a particular way, yet experience absolutely no anxiety if I am certain that I will successfully convey the desired image. Only if there is some doubt that I will make the desired impression will I feel socially anxious.

We will assume that, whenever people attempt to manage their impressions before others, they hold expectancies regarding the likelihood that they will be successful at conveying the desired image. Borrowing from Bandura's (1977) notion of self-efficacy, I will call the subjective probability of conveying any particular image of oneself to others *self-presentational efficacy*. Being a probability, one's self-presentational efficacy may range from .00 to 1.00. When one's self-presentational efficacy is .00, the individual sees absolutely no possibility of making the impressions he or she is motivated to convey; in this instance—such as when I have clearly made a fool of myself—the likelihood of experiencing social anxiety is quite high, given at least minimal motivation to make a particular impression. (If I am not at all motivated to make a particular impression, I will not feel socially anxious no matter how great a fool I appear to be.) When one's self-presentational efficacy is 1.00, the individual is perfectly sure that he or she will make the desired impressions. When this is the case, there is no possibility of feeling socially anxious. Of course, in most social settings, people's perceptions of self-presentational efficacy lie between these two extremes. The theory predicts that, holding constant the motivation to make a particular impression, decreases in self-presentational efficacy will be associated with increased social anxiety.

In this chapter, we will examine the literature dealing with situational and dispositional variables that appear to influence social anxiety by affecting self-presentational efficacy. For ease of presentation, I have grouped these factors into two major classes. Self-presentational efficacy may be low because of *uncertainty* regarding the nature of the self-presentations that will have the desired effects upon other interactants. People who do not know how to make particular impressions on others are likely to doubt that they will be regarded and evaluated favorably. We will then turn to factors that lead people to expect they will not be evaluated as they desire even when they know the kinds of impressions they would like to make. People sometimes know how they would like others to perceive them, but doubt that they will successfully foster those particular impressions.

Uncertainty

When people want others to perceive and evaluate them in particular ways, they seek information regarding the most effective ways to elicit the reactions they desire. When attempting to ascertain the kinds of self-presentations that will create the desired effects, people either access such information from memory (as I recall, my date seems to like people who are witty) or glean it from cues in the current situation (this job interviewer appears to be a very conservative fellow). Whatever its source, people then use this information to modify their self-presentations in ways that they expect will produce the reactions they desire (Jones & Wortman, 1973; Schlenker, 1980). Let me reemphasize a point made in Chapter 3: Controlling one's self-presentations in order to project particular social images to others does not necessarily imply deceitfulness. Self-presentation is often simply a matter of choosing among a large set of equally veridical self-images for projection to others.

In many situations, people believe that they have sufficient information regarding how others are likely to react to various self-presentations to guide their behavior. When dealing with those they know well, for instance, people generally have a good idea of how other interactants will respond to particular behaviors and fostered impressions. A man may recognize that his coworkers appreciate his ability to tell off-color jokes whereas his parents do not.

In other situations, however, cues regarding how one should act in order to make the "right" impressions are absent, ambiguous, or contradictory, providing the individual with few clues about how he or she should respond. Without knowing others' likes, dislikes, prejudices, preferences, weaknesses, hang-ups, pet peeves, and personal characteristics, people may find it difficult to formulate a plan of response. Unable to ascertain how to make the desired impressions, the individual's perceived self-presentational efficacy is likely to be low, thus setting the stage for social anxiety. Indeed, some of the known antecedents of social anxiety appear to have their effect by creating uncertainty about how to make the desired impressions. Let us turn our attention to three classes of such factors: strangers, novel situations, and individual differences in the ability to ascertain cues regarding socially appropriate behavior.

STRANGERS

Strangers seem to have a special power to cause others to feel socially anxious. As Charles Darwin (1955) noted over 100 years ago, people are seldom shy in the presence of people they know well. This observation has been supported by Zimbardo's (1977) surveys, which show that more people report feeling shy in encounters with strangers than in any other type of social setting except "being the center of attention of a large group." Similarly, Jones and Russell (1982) report that their subjects listed "strangers" most often in their lists of shyness-producing stimuli; 78% of the respondents said that strangers made them feel shy.

By definition, strangers are individuals about whom people have minimal information. When interacting with others for the first time, we typically know little if anything about their personalities, religious and political orientations, likes and dislikes, lifestyles, occupations, interests, values, or the kinds of people they like or detest. Without such information, people may doubt that they can negotiate a successful and rewarding interaction. The chances of saying or doing something that the other person will regard negatively is increased. This may be one reason why encounters with strangers are focused initially on gathering information about one another (e.g., "Where did you go to school? What do you do? Married?"). Once enough information about the other is acquired, each interactant is able to respond more confidently.

Of course, many interactions with strangers are relatively impersonal and do not elicit a high degree of motivation to make a particular impression. Thus, uncertainty about how to respond is of little concern. At most, the individuals just want to get through such encounters without incurring any social costs, but they have little interest in being perceived in any particular fashion. In addition, many interactions with strangers are governed by roles and norms that provide a framework for how the participants are to respond. In such cases, knowledge about the stranger as an individual is of no value.

SITUATIONAL AND ROLE NOVELTY

Response uncertainty is also engendered in novel situations and in situations that are, for one reason or another, ambiguous (Buss, 1980; Jones & Russell, 1982; Phillips, 1968; Pilkonis, 1977b; Zimbardo, 1977). First is the case of situational novelty. Think back to your first dance, first date, your first formal dinner party, first job interview, first sexual experience, first day on a new job, or first public speaking engagement. Typically, people report that these kinds of novel situations are particularly anxiety-arousing.

Viewed in light of the self-presentation theory, this is not surprising. When in novel situations, people have few guidelines about how to respond. The vague prescription, "When in Rome, do as the Romans do," is of some help, but the individual mimicking others is not likely to hold high expectations of creating a positive impression. Uncertainty about how to respond raises doubts about one's ability to make desired impressions on others, thus increasing the likelihood of experiencing social anxiety.

Role novelty is another common source of self-presentational uncertainty that triggers social anxiety. Social behavior is often guided by the roles people occupy. A role is a part that a person plays within a given social context. Every person plays many different roles in the course of a typical day: employee, spouse, parent, teacher, club member, friend, supervisor, and so on. Associated with each role is a set of expectations regarding the appropriate behaviors for occupants of that role to perform and not perform. People who are in the role of kindergarten teacher are expected to display caring and nurturant behavior toward the children in their charge, be able to teach young children effectively, and refrain from engaging in "bad" behaviors in front of the children. People occupying the role of "construction worker" or "prostitute" would be expected to engage in entirely different sets of behaviors and convey very different kinds of self-images, many of which are diametrically opposed to those encompassed by the role of "kindergarten teacher."

Role novelty occurs when people find themselves in roles they have not previously occupied. When playing new roles, people may be unsure which behaviors are appropriate for the role and/or how to perform the behaviors they perceive to be appropriate. In addition, they may be concerned about their ability to *appear* to be playing the role appropriately. Upon getting his first job teaching in a university, a friend of mine became temporarily obsessed with appearing to be a college professor. He was quite afraid that he did not give off the impression of being a professor (as opposed to a student) and went to various extremes to play the new role as perfectly as possible. Since people are often negatively evaluated and sanctioned when they do not conform to role demands, the uncertainty caused by role novelty may cause people in new roles to experience a certain degree of social anxiety.

Adolescence is a particularly insecure, awkward, and anxiety-ridden period in many people's lives. Studies of social anxiety across the lifespan suggest that junior high school students are more likely to label themselves "shy" than any other group in American society. Part of the traumatic impact of adolescence may be traced to the fact that during the teenage years adolescents first occupy a large number of new, adult-oriented roles. For the first time in their lives, most young people get a job, have their first date, take on responsibilities in school and civic organizations and, in general, are forced to behave like adults rather than children. The occupation of new roles, often without sufficient training and preparation, results in uncertainty about how the roles should be performed and doubts that one will perform the roles successfully. Role novelty is not limited to adolescence. Anytime people take on new roles, they may experience increased social anxiety in situations in which those novel roles are relevant.

AMBIGUITY

Similarly, social anxiety tends to be experienced more in ambiguous and unstructured social settings, ones in which the "rules" regarding how to behave are not immediately obvious (Phillips, 1968; Pilkonis, 1977b; Zimbardo, 1977). As long as it is clear how one should act in a given social encounter, the participants can go about the task of trying to act in those ways. But, when an occasional monkey wrench is thrown into the interaction machinery, ambiguity, uncertainty, and anxiety are likely to occur.

Uncertainty may occur when other interactants break implicit rules of social behavior, leaving everyone in the position of having to figure out how best to proceed under the circumstances. I'm sure the reader has been in encounters in which another interactant derailed the entire conversation by responding inappropriately. For example, one person in an interaction may invoke norms to which other interactants are unwilling or unable to respond. In our culture, there is a norm of reciprocity (Gouldner, 1960) that surrounds the disclosure of personal information. When one person discloses personal information about him- or herself, others are implicitly expected to reciprocate by disclosing information about themselves (Jourard, 1964). However, if someone discloses too much too soon—by telling others about their confinement in a mental institution upon first meeting, for example—others interactants will regard the disclosure as inappropriate and be unwilling to reciprocate. The violation of norms (of appropriateness and reciprocity, respectively) by both parties creates a difficult situation in which there are few cues about how best to respond.

Similarly, when others behave in an unexpected or socially inappropriate fashion, everyone in the encounter is spun into an ambiguous situation. When one participant performs an embarrassing action, for instance, others present may become uneasy because they do not know how to respond without further complicating the situation (Goffman, 1967). Should they ignore the impropriety? Such a tack is possible if the infraction is not too flagrant. Should they dismiss it with a laugh or light-hearted remark? Should they call the offending individual to account for his or her action? Uncertain about how to respond in a way that saves face for themselves, the offender, and everyone present, people in such a situation may feel socially anxious (Miller, 1979).

SELF-MONITORING

Uncertainty about how best to respond is particularly a problem for individuals who are less sensitive to the kinds of social cues that indicate which responses are socially appropriate and which are not. To the degree that interpersonal encounters are mediated by the impressions the participants form of one another, effective interactants must be sensitive to how others are perceiving and interpreting their behavior, be able to discern which behaviors are most appropriate for the encounter, and then attempt to put this information to use to facilitate a smooth encounter and the projection of appropriate social images. Failure to monitor and control one's responses is likely to result in the projection of impressions that others deem undesirable, in negative evaluations and reactions from others, and in a stilted, awkward, and aversive interaction for all participants, but especially for the offending individual.

Social psychologists have recently become interested in differences in people's ability and willingness to monitor and control their social behavior as a function of situational cues—a characteristic that has been called *self-monitoring* (Snyder, 1974, 1979). A self-monitoring individual is one who, "out of a concern for social appropriateness, is particularly sensitive to the expression and self-presentation of others in social situations and uses these cues as guidelines for monitoring [observing and controlling] his own self-presentation" (Snyder, 1974, p. 528). High self-monitors are sensitive to cues regarding appropriate demeanor, have the ability to adjust their behavior to the contingencies of particular encounters, and use this ability to control how they come across to others. Low self-monitors, on the other hand, are not as sensitive to social cues regarding appropriate behavior and self-presentation, are not as capable of controlling the impressions others form of them, and attempt to manage their impressions less often than high self-monitors. Low self-monitors may be as expressive as highs, but their expressiveness primarily reflects their internal thoughts and feelings and derives less from socially strategic attempts to control how they are perceived in social settings.

Snyder (1974) developed a 25-item Self-Monitoring Scale to measure people's proclivity for self-monitoring. As the nature of the construct would suggest, people who score high on the Self-Monitoring Scale are more likely to rely on situational cues about how to behave and more likely to seek social comparison information about how others are responding (Snyder, 1974). They also turn more often to others for guidelines about how to cope with unfamiliar situations. In addition, high self-monitors are more sensitive to the messages hidden in others' nonverbal behavior and more successful at "reading" others' emotions from their expressions. Research by Geizer et al. (1977) found that high self-monitors were more accurate at identifying the truthful contestant on videotapes of the television show "To Tell the Truth." High self-monitors also pay more attention to and are better able to remember information about those they meet (Berscheid, Graziano, Monson, & Dermer, 1976). Such information provides guidelines about how to obtain the reactions they desire from others. Finally, research has shown that high self-monitoring individuals are more successful at tailoring their behavior and self-presentations to the contingencies of the particular situation in which they find themselves (Arkin, Gabrenya, Appelman, & Cochrane, 1979; Miller & Schlenker, 1978; Snyder & Monson, 1975). This is not to say that people who score low in self-monitoring never monitor and control their social behaviors, only that they do it less often. Given that high self-monitors are more responsive to situational cues regarding appropriate behavior, it might be expected that social anxiety is related to individual differences in self-monitoring.

The hypothesized relationships between self-monitoring and social anxiety are complex since self-monitoring is defined by a *set* of psychological characteristics. Different aspects of self-monitoring would be predicted to bear different relationships to social anxiety. To compound the complexity, recent investigations of the internal structure of the Self-Monitoring Scale have shown that it taps several relatively distinct attributes that do not perfectly match the original conceptualization of self-monitoring (Briggs, Cheek, & Buss, 1980; Gabrenya & Arkin, 1980; Leary, Silver, Schlenker, & Darby, 1982). In fact, several researchers have advocated a reconceptualization of the trait and the development of new measures (Lennox & Wolfe, 1982). Even so, existing data provide us with some insight into the role of certain aspects of self-monitoring in social anxiety.

One factor obtained in factor analyses of the Self-Monitoring Scale reflects self-monitors' tendency to observe and control their behavior depending upon the nature of the situation. Since we may assume that the tendency to monitor and control one's behavior arises from a motivation to do and say the "right" things, a positive correlation between this factor and social anxiety would be expected. Indeed, the tendency to monitor and control one's behavior correlates positively with measures of social anxiety and shyness (Briggs et al., 1980; Gabrenya & Arkin, 1980).

A second factor found in analyses of the scale reflects respondents' self-perceived "acting ability"—the ability to control one's expressive behaviors in the way a good actor does. Since such an ability constitutes a specific, adaptive social skill that should increase the person's confidence that he or she can make impressions they desire upon others, it should correlate negatively with social anxiety, which it does (Briggs et al., 1980; Gabrenya & Arkin, 1980). In short, specific components of self-monitoring correlate with social anxiety in a manner predicted by the self-presentation explanation described in Chapter 3.

PROVIDING SCRIPTS FOR THE SOCIALLY ANXIOUS

Social anxiety is heightened in situations that are novel, unstructured, and ambiguous, in interactions with strangers, and for individuals who are less adept at monitoring and controlling their self-presentations. In each of these instances, the individual is likely to lack a cogent plan or script for responding. A plan is a general problem-solving strategy aimed toward the accomplishment of goals, and a script represents sequences of specific behaviors aimed toward goal accomplishment (e.g., Landau & Goldfried, 1981). Uncertainty about how to respond and about the best self-presentations to foster in a given encounter results from not having viable social plans and/or scripts to guide one's behavior. When people do not have confidence in their plans or scripts for an encounter, they are likely to doubt that they will be able to make the impressions upon others they would like to and, thus, expect to be perceived and evaluated less favorably than they desire.

What this suggests is that social anxiety caused by response uncertainty can be reduced by providing people with the information they need to formulate appropriate plans and scripts (Schlenker & Leary, 1982). In many cases, simply briefing people regarding what they can expect in novel situations should reduce uncertainty and social anxiety. Knowing what to expect on one's first date, on a job interview, at a convention, in an oral examination, or at a business meeting should provide rough but useful guidelines. Similarly, teaching people how they should behave in a novel situation or role should reduce uncertainty. Much of the anguish of adolescence could be minimized if parents and teachers took it upon themselves to prepare children and adolescents for new roles and situations. Too often we learn our social scripts and interpersonal skills through trial and error.

Pilkonis (1977b) suggests that dispositionally "shy" people could be taught to set their own "interaction agenda" in ambiguous and unstructured social settings. Rather than waiting insecurely to respond to cues provided by others, people could learn a number of all-purpose scripts for use in encounters in which response uncertainty would otherwise be quite high. By taking an active role in structuring the encounter, the individual is able to respond more confidently. If one thinks about individuals who seem most at ease conversing with strangers, it can be seen that they are not generally performing any great interpersonal feat. Rather, they are simply providing their own structure to the conversation by asking questions or directing the conversational topics. Their confidence and poise arise from the fact that *they are in control.* These same individuals often become reticent and inhibited when they are not in control of the encounter and must respond in accordance with others' scripts.

For those individuals who "never know what to say" in unstructured and ambiguous encounters, one solution would be to teach them to structure the situation in ways that best suit them—to impose their own, preplanned script upon the interaction. For example, they could be encouraged to follow the implicit plan of finding out as much as possible about other interactants. Stipulating such a goal in advance serves several functions. First, it provides a framework for responding in unstructured situations—when in doubt, the individual can always put this sort of all-purpose plan into action. Armed with a specific plan, the person will never be paralyzed by social uncertainty. Second, this particular mode of response (i.e., finding out about others) keeps the focus of attention off oneself and onto other interactants, while allowing the anxious individual to acquire information about the other that will allow them to respond in the most facilitative fashion possible. Finally, the individual who provides structure to otherwise awkward interactions will generally be regarded favorably. In particular the tack of trying to learn about other interactants presents one in a very favorable light. As Dale Carnegie noted (1936, p. 88), the person you are talking to "is a hundred times more interested in himself and his wants and his problems than he is in you and your problems." Interactants who show interest in others are regarded as friendly, sociable, and likeable.

Counselors and clinicians who deal with socially anxious clients might try teaching them strategies that will help to reduce the anxiety born of uncertainty. Along these lines, one self-help paperback that suggests ways of overcoming shyness presents several all-purpose scripts for conversations (Powell, 1979). Research is needed that assesses the effectiveness of various techniques designed to teach people to be more facile at responding in unstructured, ambiguous, and novel situations.

UNCERTAINTY IN CONTINGENT AND NONCONTINGENT ENCOUNTERS

All of the examples I have used when discussing the impact of response or self-presentational uncertainty on social anxiety have involved contingent, conversational encounters. This is because uncertainty is a much greater problem in contingent than noncontingent encounters. In most (but not all) noncontingent social settings, such as plays, speeches, concerts, and other public performances before audiences, people's actions are guided by very explicit plans, whether they be speeches, scripts, or musical scores. These prepared scripts are generally not open to extensive revision during the course of the performance, so that people in noncontingent encounters are unlikely to have doubts about how they should behave during the encounter itself. (They may, however, doubt their ability to execute the script successfully, as will be discussed below.) Uncertainty will result only if the performer either forgets part of a memorized script, in which case absolute uncertainty and intense anxiety will occur, or attempts to ad-lib or improvise.

For most noncontingent encounters, uncertainty about how best to respond occurs *before* the encounter itself, while the plan is being devised. For example, a person preparing a speech may not be sure of the best way to influence his audience and may feel apprehensive while writing the text. Having written the speech, however, there should be no uncertainty about how to act although, again, the speaker may doubt that the speech will be well received.

Since one's behavior in a *contingent* encounter is modified on the basis of what other interactants say and do, uncertainty about how to respond at any given moment is more likely and thus the likelihood that one will experience social anxiety also increases. In addition, people who characteristically have difficulty discerning how to behave should be more bothered by contingent than noncontingent encounters.

Self-Perceived Ability to Control Impressions

Ascertaining the most efficacious self-presentations for a given encounter is only the first step in conveying a particular impression of oneself to others. Once a person has an idea of the kinds of impressions likely to result in valued outcomes, he or she must successfully convey those images. People may know how they should respond in order to obtain the evaluations and reactions they desire, but continue to hold a low expectancy of actually doing so. Believing that they do not possess the characteristics, abilities, accomplishments, or resources to successfully claim the image, such individuals are likely to feel socially anxious (Schlenker & Leary, 1982).

I am reminded of an unassuming freshman advisee I had a few years ago. Coming from a small, predominately lower class high school, she found herself at college with a high percentage of status-minded students from wealthy families. She perceived that a certain set of self-images was needed to gain acceptance into the mainstream of campus social life, but initially doubted that she could foster such self-images successfully. She had no previous exposure to the prevailing values, behavior, or dress of many of the students. Her self-perceived inability to project the self-presentations that she believed were needed resulted in considerable insecurity and social anxiety. However, after a relatively rapid period of transformation in clothing and behavior that rendered her indistinguishable from other students, she developed increased confidence in her ability to convey the kinds of impressions others would value. She continued to recognize that she was only playing a part, so to speak, but believed that she was playing it successfully. Although she sometimes felt uncomfortable behaving in ways contrary to her own standards and beliefs, she seldom experienced social anxiety thereafter. This case demonstrates one unfortunate concomitant of evaluation apprehension—increased conformity to norms—but, more central to our present discussion, it suggests that doubts in one's ability to convey the kinds of impressions one is motivated to convey results in social anxiety. Conversely, the belief that one can successfully project certain social images reduces social anxiety, whether or not the projected images are consistent with one's own self-concept.

A least-of-evils choice is faced by the individual who is motivated to make particular impressions but doubts he or she will be able to do so. Desired social outcomes may not be forthcoming unless an attempt is made to make the desired impressions, but the individual holds a low expectancy of doing so. Since people are evaluated negatively when they do not possess the characteristics that legitimately permit them to claim an image, they generally do not try to appear in ways that might be contradicted by what others know or are likely to find out about them (Baumeister & Jones, 1978; Schlenker, 1975). My student was, in a sense, "lucky." Since no one on campus knew anything about her, she was able to create whatever public image she desired.

A number of situational and dispositional factors appear to influence social anxiety by affecting people's level of subjective confidence in their abilities to convey the kinds of impressions they are motivated to project to others. In this section, we will examine several such variables, including self-evaluation, the expertise and ability of others in the social encounter, aversive experiences in past social settings, the number of coperformers with whom one is performing in a noncontingent encounter, the individual's self-perceived level of physical attractiveness and social skill, Type A personality, and self-presentational predicaments.

SELF-EVALUATION

Perhaps the most replicated finding in the social anxiety literature is the negative relationship between social anxiety and self-evaluation. Self-esteem has been found to be negatively correlated with measures of shyness (Cheek & Buss, 1981; Cheek, 1982; Zimbardo, 1977), communication apprehension (Huntley, 1969; McCroskey, 1977), social avoidance and distress (Clark & Arkowitz, 1975), social anxiousness (Cheek, 1982; Leary, 1983a; Leavy, 1980) and audience anxiousness (Cheek, 1982; Leary, 1983a). It has also been found that highly socially anxious people make more self-deprecating statements about themselves than do less anxious people (Cacioppo et al., 1979; Glass et al., 1982; Smith & Breck, 1982), and that low self-esteem people report greater levels of shyness and anxiety in laboratory conversations than do high self-esteem individuals (Leavy, 1980). The relationship between self-esteem and social anxiety is undisputed and provides the basis for one of the cognitive approaches to social anxiety discussed in Chapter 2.

As I observed earlier, however, low self-esteem is neither necessary nor sufficient to produce social anxiety. Low self-evaluation should result in social anxiety only to the degree that it leads people to anticipate that *others* will also evaluate them unfavorably. In most instances, individuals who perceive some aspect of themselves negatively will assume that others will rate them unfavorably as well. However, *if* one believes that there is little chance that self-perceived deficiencies will be detected by others, social anxiety should not occur. It is possible to imagine a situation in which a person with low self-esteem believes that the other interactants in a particular encounter will evaluate him or her favorably. Will the person feel socially anxious? The self-presentational model of social anxiety says "no," since the individual has a high sense of self-presentational efficacy in the encounter regardless of his or her self-evaluation. Thus, self-evaluation is related to social anxiety only indirectly via the individual's assumptions regarding how he or she is perceived and evaluated by others.

In addition, low self-evaluations are related to social anxiety only to the extent that the negative self-perceptions are relevant to important personal attributes that may be evaluated by others (Sutton-Simon & Goldfried, 1979). Negative self-perceptions on attributes that are not open to scrutiny by others should not result in social anxiety.

STANDARDS FOR SELF-EVALUATION

People learn to evaluate themselves and their behavior based on past reactions of significant other people (Bandura, 1977). Over time, people internalize standards that are then used for self-evaluation. We tend to think that such standards are learned primarily during childhood, but in fact people may internalize others' standards for self-evaluation whenever they do not possess a standard relevant to a particular behavioral domain. An adult may begin to assess his or her technique on the tennis court after learning the appropriate criteria and standards for evaluation from the tennis instructor, for example. Once standards are internalized, people react with approval and satisfaction when their behavior meets or exceeds the relevant standard, but with disapproval and dissatisfaction when it does not (cf. Bandura, 1977; Carver, 1979).

People hold a vast number of standards for self-evaluation, each of which is relevant to a particular behavioral domain. A woman might have standards for evaluating her performance on tests (and perhaps different standards for different courses), her moral behavior, her athletic prowess, her job performance, and so on. She receives implicit and explicit feedback regarding her behavioral performances in each of these domains and compares it to the relevant standard.

In the same manner, people seem to hold standards for assessing the quality or effectiveness of their self-presentations. When people attempt to convey particular impressions of themselves, they assess the effectiveness of the attempt through the feedback they receive from others. Thus, the relevant feedback for assessing one's self-presentations are the perceived or imagined impression-relevant reactions of others (Schlenker & Leary, 1982). People appear to compare the reactions they believe they are receiving from others to their internal standards. Although no research has specifically examined such standards, their presence can be inferred from the fact that people often conclude they have made "good" impressions on others or sometimes believe they have made "bad" impressions. The evaluation of their self-presentations implies the existence of standards for making these sorts of judgments.

People differ greatly in the stringency of their standards. One only need observe students receiving test grades. Of two students receiving B's on the test, one may be delighted, while the other is crushed. The difference in their reactions lies in the level of their standards of self-evaluation. Likewise, people's standards for evaluating their self-presentations differ. Some people hold very high standards and require very favorable impression-relevant reactions from others in order to be satisfied and self-approving. Others' standards are lower. They require only minimally approving feedback from others in order to feel satisfied with the effectiveness of their self-presentations.

This suggests a link between personal standards and social anxiety: All other things being equal, the higher one's standards for assessing self-presentational efficacy, the higher the likelihood of experiencing social anxiety. A person whose standards are excessively high may often feel socially anxious, not because others' reactions were objectively unfavorable but because their reactions did not come up to his or her standards (see Bandura, 1969). In many instances, others may judge the individual quite favorably, but, in the actor's eyes, not favorably enough. In line with this, Zimbardo (1981b) notes that many instances of shyness are precipitated by the adoption of exaggerated criteria for self-evaluation. Nichols (1974) observed that highly socially anxious individuals tend to hold very rigid concepts of what constitutes appropriate and inappropriate behavior.

When people evaluate themselves, they often compare themselves to others. In most instances, the most useful and informative comparisons are those made in reference to others who are similar to oneself on the relevant dimension (Festinger, 1954). Comparison of oneself with those who are clearly far superior or inferior does not provide the individual with very useful information about his abilities and outcomes. For example, a person giving a speech in public would most likely evaluate his or her speech and the audience reactions it elicits to those of other speakers of approximately equal ability. Not much is gained by comparing one's speaking ability with either a world renowned orator or a person with a speech disorder.

Unfortunately, people sometimes evaluate themselves in reference to models who are highly regarded for excellence in the relevant domain, thus employing standards that are unrealistically high (Bandura, 1969). A teenage girl who compares herself with a fashion model or movie actress—even a teenage one—is likely to feel dissatisfied with her appearance, poise, and social skill. Her attempts at social interaction will always fall far short of the standards she holds. As a result, she is likely to feel anxious when contemplating her "shortcomings."

Interestingly, people who are high in fear of negative evaluation (which as we have seen is associated with social anxiety) prefer to compare themselves, when possible, with those of *lesser* ability when their sense of competence is threatened (Friend & Gilbert, 1973). Comparing oneself to those who are worse-off on the dimension in question allows the individual who fears negative evaluations to feel better about himself or herself by contrast. In other words, one way to reduce apprehension about being regarded unfavorably is to lower one's standards.

Although it might be expected that people who have experienced a high degree of social success in the past would be more confident and less anxious as time goes on, such is not necessarily the case. People tend to revise their standards upward as they experience success. The result is that they are no longer satisfied with the earlier level of performance and outcomes. The actress who, as a beginner, was happy just to remember her lines, is now not satisfied with anything less than a truly outstanding performance and rave reviews. The young man who was once delighted just to get a date now feels he has failed if he doesn't knock women off their feet. The result of constantly revising one's standards upward with success is that many individuals who, by all indications, should be confident and self-assured continue to experience a great deal of social anxiety. The evaluations and reactions they receive from others seldom meet their high standards. This may explain why some television personalities describe themselves as shy despite their success and public acceptance (Leary & Schlenker, 1981; Zimbardo, 1977).

Counselors and clinicians often see clients whose personal distress derives from excessively high standards for self-evaluation. Therapies based upon rational-emotive and cognitive restructuring approaches are applicable in such cases (see Chapter 2). Clients can be shown that their unhappiness and anxiety is a function of their unrealistic expectations and can then be taught more facilitative ways to view themselves and their social worlds.

EXPERTISE AND ABILITY OF OTHER INTERACTANTS

I mentioned earlier that people often report feeling shy when interacting with those they perceive as competent, expert, or highly skilled (Jones & Russell, 1982; Zimbardo, 1977). At the time, I attributed this in part to the fact that people are often more highly motivated to make an impression on those they hold in high esteem than those they do not. A second possibility is that this kind of audience is more likely to make people doubt that they can suitably impress them. It is no surprise that people who are seen as knowledgeable, competent, or skilled would be regarded as harder to please. Not only will I be more highly motivated to impress them, I may also be more likely to doubt that I will do so. Of course, the dimension on which the others are highly regarded must be relevant to the kinds of impressions I wish to make in order for their expertise to affect my social anxiety. I may not be particularly nervous singing in front of a group of highly skilled butchers, but might feel nervous if my audience was composed of professional opera singers (Knight & Borden, 1978).

An experiment by Brown and Garland (1972) showed that people will even sacrifice monetary incentives to avoid projecting undesirable images of themselves to competent others. Subjects were told that they would be paid to sing in front of an audience that would evaluate their singing voices. They would be paid at the rate of 1¢ for every five seconds they sang and could sing for as long or as short a time as they wished. (Although this may sound like a meager amount of money, it amounts to $7.20 per hour.) Half of the subjects were told that the evaluating audience consisted of poor singers, whereas the other half believed that they would sing to excellent singers. As expected, subjects sang for significantly less time (and, thus, collected less money) when their audience was ostensibly composed of excellent rather than poor singers. We've already discussed Knight and Borden's (1978) finding that people report greater anxiety when they sing before those with high rather than low musical ability (Chapter 4).

Although no studies have been conducted to examine this effect in contingent kinds of encounters, I would expect that people feel more socially anxious when conversing with those who are highly socially skilled. Some people we deal with are superbly poised, articulate, and otherwise socially adept, whereas others are not. It seems likely that most people regard highly socially skilled individuals as harder to please and expect to make less favorable impressions upon them. It would be easy to experimentally test the hypothesis that people experience greater social anxiety when interacting with those to whom they think they pale by comparison.

Apparently, most people think that knowledgeable, competent, and skilled individuals hold higher standards for evaluating other people, are harder to please, and are less tolerant of below average performances than less competent individuals. As a result, people are more likely to experience social anxiety in those encounters in which they are motivated to make particular impressions upon such individuals.

PAST EXPERIENCES

Every person is his or her own biographer, duly recording—although occasionally with embellishments and distortions—his or her experiences in life. People's recollections of past occurrences can have a major impact on the way they deal with similar events in the future. In particular, a history of past successes in social encounters leads people to expect positive social experiences in the future, whereas a history of social failures (whether real or perceived) leads to expectations of negative social experiences. People who have had unsuccessful, punishing, awkward, and otherwise aversive experiences in social settings in the past may then greet the prospect of subsequent encounters with some trepidation. Such experiences lead people to doubt that they can make the kinds of impressions on others that will result in desired reactions from them, precipitating social anxiety.

Many people can point to a single, specific event or series of events in their past that led them to first doubt their social competence. In many cases, the memory of a *single* traumatic experience remains powerful enough to trigger anxiety when similar situations are encountered (Zimbardo, 1977). In other instances, people's feelings of anxiety may derive from a *series* of aversive experiences over a period of time. For example, a good predictor of whether or not a person will experience audience anxiety while giving a speech is the sheer number of rewarding experiences he or she has had in such situations in the past (Paivio & Lambert, 1959). People who have had a large number of rewarding social experiences are less prone to audience anxiety than those with fewer rewarding experiences.

The classical conditioning model of social anxiety discussed in Chapter 2 is applicable here. Viewed from a social learning perspective, classical conditioning occurs when people associate certain situations with positive or negative outcomes (Bandura, 1969, 1977). Past aversive episodes lead the person to expect aversive consequences in the future, heightening the likelihood of social anxiety.

NUMBER OF CO-PERFORMERS

Although the prospect of speaking or performing in front of an audience is anxiety-arousing for much of the population, the aversiveness of the experience is diminished when people perform as members of a group rather than alone. The presence of co-performers reduces social anxiety.

In a field study by Jackson and Latane (1981, Study 2), college students participated in a Greek-Week talent show in front of an audience of approximately 2500 at a major state university. The number of performers in the various musical, dancing, and comedy acts ranged from 1 to 10, allowing Jackson and Latane to examine the relationship between the number of coperformers in one's act and the individual's level of social anxiety. As expected, results demonstrated an inverse relationship. The greater the number of coperformers, the less nervous each performer felt. As with increases in the size of the audience discussed earlier, more coperformers had an increasingly smaller effect on performers' anxiety as the size of the group in the act increased. That is, although performers felt much less nervous when they performed with four than two other people, there was not much difference in the nervousness of performers performing in groups of ten versus seven, for example.

An earlier study also demonstrates the effects of the number of coperformers on overt manifestations of social anxiety. A common indication that a person is very anxious is an increase in speech disfluencies, such as hesitating, stammering, stuttering, repeating oneself, and using an oversupply of "ahs" and "uhs." In a study of chronic stutterers, Barber (1939) showed that people stuttered less when they read a passage in unison with others rather than alone. The difference in stuttering between the conditions was quite pronounced: Those reading alone stuttered on an average of 21% of the words, whereas those who read with three coperformers stuttered on only 1% of the words!

These and similar findings clearly show that social anxiety decreases as the number of coperformers increases. But, why? It may be that when people perform with others, they perceive that the audience's attention is divided among all performers. As a result, coperforming reduces people's concerns that they will personally make unfavorable impressions upon members of the audience. The solo speaker or performer stands or falls on the merits of his or her own performance. By performing in a group, the self-presentational risks are generally lowered. Although one's sense of accomplishment for superior performances is diminished somewhat when the performance is a group endeavor, this is more than enough to offset the potential negative repercussions of inferior performances for many people. Not only are the individual performer's weaknesses less easily discernable and possibly compensated for by others in the group, but the responsibility for an unsatisfactory performance can be distributed among all participants. It is never pleasant to have one's group "bomb out" on stage, but the individual performers may at least take consolation in the fact that the audience can usually not determine who was really responsible for the bad showing. Poor performances are simply less devastating to one's public image (and likely one's *self*-image) when people perform in groups.

An exception to this general principle arises when people believe they are personally capable of a satisfactory performance, but anticipate that their coperformers are not as skilled, talented, or prepared as themselves. In such cases, the individual may expect that coperformers' poor performances will make the entire group, including him- or herself, look bad. In this instance, social anxiety is not likely to be decreased by increasing numbers of incompetent coperformers.

PHYSICAL ATTRACTIVENESS

Despite clichés such as "You can't judge a book by its cover" and "Beauty is only skin deep," people's impressions and evaluations of others *are* heavily influenced by the other's level of physical attractiveness. Attractive persons are generally assumed to rank higher than less attractive persons on virtually every positive personality characteristic. They are assumed to be more warm, kind, responsive, interesting, poised, sociable, modest, strong, outgoing, socially adept, and humorous (Berscheid & Walster, 1974; Snyder, Tanke, & Berscheid, 1977). Attractive individuals are also assumed to have more successful marriages and to lead more fulfilling lives (Dion, Berscheid, & Walster, 1972). Similarly, research by Dion (1972) showed that adults were more likely to judge children who misbehaved as characteristically antisocial if the child was unattractive rather than attractive.

Not only are attractive individuals liked better than less attractive ones (e.g., Walster, Aronson, Abrahams, & Rottman, 1966), in addition people respond more favorably to them. Barocas and Karoly (1972) found that males provided attractive women with more social reinforcement and desired their friendship more. In a study in which men interacted with women over an intercom, Snyder et al. (1977) showed that men who thought their conversation partners were attractive were rated more sociable, warm, independent, outgoing, humorous, bold, and socially skilled than men who thought they were talking with a less attractive woman. Other research has demonstrated that people evaluate authors' writings more highly when they believe the author is attractive rather than unattractive (Landy & Sigall, 1974), and are more easily influenced by attractive than unattractive others (Mills & Aronson, 1965).

Now to return to social anxiety. Given the emphasis that is commonly placed on physical appearance, people who perceive themselves as relatively unattractive may hold a lower sense of self-presentational efficacy than people who see themselves as attractive. They will be more likely to doubt that they will create sufficiently favorable impressions upon others and be evaluated and treated as they desire. As a result, people who view themselves as unattractive might be on the average more likely to experience social anxiety when they are motivated to make a favorable impression. Empirical data bearing upon this hypothesis is scanty and equivocal. On one hand, Pilkonis (1977b) found that experimenters, confederates, and trained observers rated shy subjects (identified by the Stanford Shyness Survey) as significantly less physically attractive than nonshy subjects. However, Cheek and Buss (1981) found no differences in observers' attractiveness ratings for women classified as high versus low in shyness on the basis of their Shyness Scale.

In light of the emphasis placed on appearance in social encounters, it would be surprising if self-perceived attractiveness was found to be unrelated to one's subjective probability of making a good overall impression on others. After all, why do we go to such lengths to make ourselves look better? It may be, however, that self-perceived attractiveness is most strongly related to social anxiety in *cross-sex* encounters. People are generally more concerned with how they look to those of the other sex than to those of their own sex. In support of this notion, I have unpublished data showing that heterosocial anxiousness (social anxiousness experienced in encounters with those of the other sex) is negatively correlated with self-ratings of physical attractiveness.

If a link between self-perceived physical appearance and social anxiety is substantiated by future research, it suggests that one mode of treatment for some socially anxious individuals might be to assist them in improving their appearance. Most people's appearances can be enhanced somewhat via a new hairstyle, better-fitting clothes, improved posture, and so on. In addition, teaching clients to use certain expressive behaviors, such as smiling, head-nodding, and eye contact, should improve their overall attractiveness to others (see Holstein, Goldstein, & Bem, 1971; Kleinke, Staneski, & Berger, 1975). In more extreme cases, some psychotherapists recommend cosmetic surgery for clients who are bothered by their facial appearance (Berscheid & Walster, 1974). In each case, these sorts of enhancements might be expected to improve the individual's attractiveness, increase his or her confidence in his or her ability to make good impressions, result in more favorable reactions from other interactants, and reduce social anxiety.

PERCEIVED SOCIAL SKILL DIFFICULTIES

The social skills model of social anxiety discussed in Chapter 2 posits that social anxiety often results from a deficit in important social skills. However, as we saw, it has been difficult to identify specific social deficiencies among highly socially anxious people. We are now ready to show how the social skills model fits into the broader self-presentation theory of social anxiety.

According to the self-presentation approach, social skill deficits affect social anxiety indirectly by leading people who see themselves as socially deficient to anticipate failing at their attempts to convey particular impressions of themselves to others. Believing that one lacks important social skills—such as a sense of humor, the ability to carry on a conversation without faltering, or public speaking ability—may lead the individual to conclude that he or she is unlikely to make a favorable impression or be evaluated positively in those social settings in which such skills are needed.

It is important to note that, according to this view, the central factor is not a deficit in social skills per se, but a *self-perceived* social inadequacy. Even horribly unskilled individuals are unlikely to feel anxious if they fail to recognize their social limitations. On the other hand, some highly skilled and socially poised people may become socially anxious when they doubt that they can handle a particular encounter. People with low self-esteem, for example, may underestimate their ability to deal effectively with others and may experience social anxiety even though they are socially adept.

The counseling approach for individuals with self-perceived social difficulties depends upon the veridicality of the client's self-perception. If the client is cognizant of a real social deficit that does in fact interfere with his or her ability to navigate certain kinds of social channels, social skills training is the treatment of choice (Bellack & Hersen, 1979; Curran, 1977). The client can be taught the necessary interpersonal skills through the techniques outlined in Chapter 2. Of course, the counselor must be sure that changes in the client's social behavior are accompanied by corresponding changes in self-evaluation. It is entirely possible for a client who has now learned effective ways of handling social encounters to continue to perceive himself or herself as socially deficient.

If the social skill deficit is more *imagined* than real, social skills training is likely to be of limited effectiveness, except perhaps as an indirect way of building the client's self-confidence in social settings. In the case of imagined social and personal deficiencies, steps must be taken to help the client modify inaccurate self-conceptions.

TYPE A

This section is admittedly speculative. I felt that the unexamined link between Type A and social anxiety was sufficiently provocative to be included nonetheless.

Type A refers to a response style characterized by a high degree of competitive achievement striving, an exaggerated sense of time urgency (i.e., always feeling that one does not have enough time to get everything done), and high aggressiveness in response to frustration (Glass, 1977). Individuals who possess these characteristics to a relatively high degree are classified as Type A; those who seldom exhibit these responses are labeled Type B. These behavioral patterns have received widespread research attention in recent years because of the finding that Type A people have at least twice the incidence of coronary heart disease as Type B's (Friedman & Rosenman, 1974). The link between Type A and heart disease is a fascinating topic but it does not concern us here. Rather, I would like to describe one study that suggests that Type A people possess characteristics that may predispose them to experience social anxiety more often than Type B people.

Brunson (1982) had Type A and Type B college students watch videotapes of a college professor discussing a student's paper with the student. Half of the subjects saw the professor convey approval to the student, whereas half saw the professor express disapproval. Subjects were then asked to rate the degree of approval-disapproval they believed the professor had expressed. Although the ratings of Type A and B subjects did not differ from one another when disapproval had been given, Type A subjects were significantly less certain that approval had been given than Type B subjects when the professor had been approving. Type A's were also found to be more likely to interpret ambiguous feedback as indicating disapproval than were Type B's.

The implication is that Type A people may fail to detect cues indicating approval from others and, thus, be less certain that others are responding favorably to them. As a result, they may strive harder to gain others' approval and acceptance (which may be partially responsible for their high achievement striving). In short, Type A people may face social situations with two response sets that increase the chances they will feel socially anxious: They are highly motivated to win others' esteem (Matthews, Helmreich, Beane, & Lucker, 1980), and they are less likely to believe that others are responding favorably to them (Brunson, 1982). Whether Type A people are actually more susceptible to feelings of social anxiety than Type B's remains an open, researchable question.

PREDICAMENTS

Each of the factors discussed in this chapter may precipitate social anxiety by reducing people's confidence in their ability to make certain kinds of impressions in a particular social setting. However, in none of the instances discussed so far has anything *in particular* happened that has clearly cast undesirable aspersions upon the individual and thus threatened the image he or she desires to project. Certain factors may lead people to believe that they will not make the impressions they desire, but nothing has happened within the encounter that has objectively and undeniably resulted in the individual coming across to others in unflattering ways.

In some situations, however, people's self-presentational plights may be much worse. Occasionally, events occur during interpersonal encounters that blatantly damage the images one or more interactants desire to project. In social psychological terms, such situations are called "predicaments"—situations in which events have undesirable implications for the kinds of images the individual has claimed or wishes to claim (Schlenker, 1980). The occurrence of a predicament usually convinces the actor that there is little chance of making the kinds of impressions he or she desired to make, making their expectation of self-presentational efficacy near or at zero. As a result, the experience of social anxiety is often quite intense.

Examples of predicaments are legion, encompassing those we often call "embarrassing" or "shameful" experiences. They range from relatively minor incidents that produce only mild and fleeting chagrin when the turn of events make the individual appear foolish, forgetful, clumsy, or in other mildly undesirable ways, to severe breaches of proper social conduct that cause irreparable damage to a person's social identity. The severity of a predicament is a function of two factors. First, the more undesirable the event that caused the predicament, the more severe the person's predicament is (Schlenker, 1980) and the greater the anxiety the person will experience. The second factor involves the person's apparent responsibility for the predicament, which may range from no responsibility to full responsibility. All other things being equal, the more responsibility the individual is seen as having for the undesirable event, the more severe the predicament and the higher the resulting level of social anxiety. Of course, the worst possible case, from the individual's perspective, is to be seen as highly responsible for a very negative occurrence, in which case social anxiety should be maximal.

Although predicaments are (thankfully) relatively rare social events, they usually induce a very high level of social anxiety when they occur. Predicaments are so highly anxiety-producing because image-threatening events make it absolutely clear to the individual that his or her public image has sustained damage; the probability of projecting the kinds of images he or she is motivated to project is near zero. The individual feels highly anxious, apprehensive, self-conscious, and flustered—the group of responses we typically label embarrassment. Viewed in this way, embarrassment is social anxiety experienced in response to a self-presentational predicament.[1]

When they find themselves in a predicament, people usually engage in remedial behaviors or "face work" in an attempt to repair their social images (Goffman, 1955, 1971; Schlenker, 1980). They may try to deny responsibility for the negative event, use excuses to minimize as best they can how responsible they appear to be for the predicament, apologize for the infraction, and/or withdraw from the encounter entirely (Schlenker, 1980). To the degree that victims of a predicament believe they were successful in reducing the severity of the predicament and repairing their public images, they should feel less socially anxious.

Summary

Once a person desires to be perceived in particular ways by others in a social setting, the belief that there is a low likelihood of conveying the desired images results in social anxiety. On one hand, the individual may be uncertain about the nature of the self-presentations that will result in the evaluations and reactions they desire to obtain. When interacting with strangers or in novel or ambiguous situations, for example, people may be unable to discern how to create the "best" impression. On the other hand, once a person knows the kinds of images he or she would like to foster, a number of factors may lead him or her to hold a low expectancy of actually doing so. Perceived self-presentational efficacy is affected by one's self-evaluation, the perceived characteristics of other interactants, past successes and failures in social situations, the number of coperformers present, perceived physical attractiveness and social skill, and self-presentational predicaments.

Note

1. When people find themselves in a predicament, they usually label their own reaction to it either "embarrassment" or "shame" (cf. Buss, 1980). The difference in peo-

ple's uses of the two terms seems to lie in the nature of the infraction that caused the predicament. If the event reflects upon the violation of *social* prescriptions regarding appropriate conduct, people tend to describe themselves as "embarrassed." The events have reflected upon the individual's personal or social attributes. However, if the predicament resulted from violations of *moral, ethical, or legal* codes, people are likely to say they are "ashamed." Because infractions resulting from the latter type of event are generally viewed more negatively by others, shame is often reported to be a more potent experience than embarrassment (Buss, 1980).

6

BEHAVIORAL CONCOMITANTS AND THEIR CONSEQUENCES

So far, we have focused primarily on antecedents of the internal, subjective experience of social anxiety. As everyone who has experienced social anxiety can attest, subjective feelings of nervousness in interpersonal encounters are often accompanied by certain behaviors that exacerbate the difficulties of the socially anxious individual. For example, when people feel socially anxious, they tend to communicate less effectively, fail to initiate conversations, act hesitant, inhibited, and awkward, and may withdraw from the encounter entirely when possible. Not only do these sorts of responses interfere with the individual's attempts to respond appropriately in the anxiety-producing situation, but they cue others into the fact that the individual is nervous and create additional concerns about one's ability to handle the encounter that, in turn, exacerbate anxiety.

For many, the behaviors that accompany episodes of social anxiety constitute a greater problem than the anxiety itself. Many people who seek counseling for social difficulties are concerned primarily with behavioral problems and only secondarily with subjective anxiety. Apparently, people differ in the degree to which they see the behavioral concomitants of social anxiety as problematic. Pilkonis (1977a) asked 100 college-age subjects who identified themselves as "shy" to rank the degree to which various subjective and behavioral aspects of shyness were a problem for them. Pilkonis interpreted the results of a cluster analysis of these rankings to show that people can be classified as "publicly" versus "privately" shy. Publicly shy subjects tended to be bothered more by public aspects of shyness, such as behaving awkwardly and failing to respond appropriately. The privately shy subjects reported that they were bothered more by the subjective cognitive and affective experience, such as their internal arousal and apprehension about being evaluated negatively. Not surprisingly, publicly shy subjects indicated that shyness was a greater personal problem for them than did privately shy subjects. When social anxiety is accompanied by overt behavioral difficulties, the individual's plight is directly observable by others present and creates additional social difficulties.

Research on the behavioral concomitants of social anxiety is of two types.[1] Some studies have compared the behavior of subjects exposed to manipulations that were designed to heighten or reduce social anxiety. Other, descriptive studies have compared the behaviors of people who were classified as "high" versus "low" in dispositional social anxiousness on the basis of one of the self-report instruments described in the Appendix. In nearly all instances, the findings of these two research strategies coincide: The behaviors observed in people exposed to experimental manipulations designed to heighten anxiety are precisely those behavioral dimensions on which high and low socially anxious people differ. This is convenient, for it allows us to discuss these bodies of research together.

The behavioral manifestations of social anxiety are quite diverse, ranging from indices of autonomic arousal to communication difficulties, social avoidance, and increased persuasibility. In my attempts to organize this portion of the social anxiety literature, it became clear that the behaviors do not all serve the same psychological and social functions for the anxious individual. Nor do they all have the same relationship to the subjective experience of anxiety itself. Some behavioral reactions appear to represent socially strategic responses, whereas others are relatively involuntary, for example. For ease of presentation and discussion, I have grouped the behavioral concomitants of social anxiety into three general categories: arousal-mediated responses, disaffilitation, and self-presentational behaviors (Leary, 1982).

Arousal-Mediated Responses

When people feel socially anxious, they tend to *act* nervous. They are likely to fidget, play with their hair, clothes, and other manipulatable objects, rub their damp hands together, lick their lips, squirm, stammer, and, in general, respond in ways that others are likely to label "nervous" (see Cheek & Buss, 1981; Pilkonis, 1977b; Murray, 1971; Zimbardo, 1977). These are examples of what I will call arousal-mediated or simply "nervous" responses—behaviors that are a direct manifestation of the anxious individual's aroused state.

Whether caused by social or nonsocial factors, anxiety is, by definition, always accompanied by arousal of the sympathetic nervous system. Sympathetic arousal effects are quite diffuse, resulting in heightened activity in some bodily systems (heartrate, respiration, blood pressure, perspiration, muscle tension) and decreased activity in others (digestion). The few studies that have taken physiological measures from socially anxious people verify that they are more autonomically aroused than nonanxious people (Borkovec et al., 1974; Leary, 1983b; Brodt & Zimbardo, 1981; see, however, Miller & Arkowitz, 1977). Many of the relatively involuntary responses of socially anxious people appear to arise partly from their high level of arousal although the empirical evidence bearing on this point is indirect.

First, a high level of anxiety is often accompanied by speech disfluencies. People who are anxious or afraid, for whatever reason, often stutter, stammer, vacilate on words, have a quivering voice, pause more frequently while speaking, and, in general, communicate less effectively (Kasl & Mahl, 1965; Mahl, 1956; Porter, 1939; Schwartz, 1976). Speech disfluencies of this kind are increased by large audiences (Porter, 1939; Siegel & Haugen, 1964), the presence of authority figures (Sheehan, Hadley, & Gould, 1967), and by unfavorable reactions from listeners (Hansen, 1955; cited in Van Riper, 1971), precisely the kinds of situations that exacerbate social anxiety. Conversely, social settings that reduce social anxiety, such as speaking or reading to children (Ramig, Krieger, & Adams, 1982) or performing with larger groups (Porter, 1939), reduce stuttering. It is important to note that changes in speech are produced by nonsocial sources of threat as well. For example, people's quality of speech is affected by the belief they are about to receive an electric shock (Murray, 1971; Van Riper, 1971).

The precise mechanism by which anxiety interferes with speaking is not fully understood. One possibility is that preoccupation with the source of the threat makes it difficult for the individual to pay sufficient attention to what he or she is saying. Instead of focusing on the ongoing interaction or on one's prepared text, for example, the socially anxious person may be preoccupied with threats of impending social doom. The nervous partier at a cocktail hour may dwell on how badly he must be coming across to others, on self-perceived social deficiencies, and on others' (imagined) negative evaluations of him. This phenomenon has been shown to debilitate test-anxious students' performance on exams (Mandler & Watson, 1966; Wine, 1971).[2] Self-deprecating and worrisome thoughts intrude into the individual's awareness and block full attention to the immediate situation.

Ironically, a second possible explanation of anxiety's effects on speech posits precisely the opposite mechanism. Stuttering may result from paying *too much* attention to what one is saying (Kamhi & McOsker, 1982). In a relaxed and friendly conversation, participants do not carefully plan or monitor precisely what they say. However, when evaluative overtones are salient, they may monitor their speech more closely and often too closely. Paying close conscious attention to actions that are normally performed "mindlessly"—without a great deal of conscious thought—disrupts the performance of the action (Baumeister, in press; Langer & Weinman, 1981). A good example is the skilled pianist who, if she concentrated on every finger movement while playing a well-rehearsed piece, would find her performance severely disrupted. Similarly, if you have ever spoken into a public address system in an auditorium or gymnasium and suddenly become aware of your voice bouncing back at you, you may have experienced the verbal disruptions that accompany overattention to one's speech. It is difficult to speak smoothly while listening to yourself.

Strictly speaking, neither of the two explanations of speaking difficulties just described posit an arousal-mediated mechanism; these hypotheses are based on cognitive and attentional processes. A third explanation is that arousal interferes with normal breathing. If you have ever tried to explain something to someone after strenuous exercise, such as running up four flights of stairs, you have experienced the effects of being out of breath on speaking. Although socially anxious people do not breathe like athletes in oxygen debt, anxiety does result in shorter, faster respiration. Schwartz (1976) presents evidence that stress produces tension in the throat that prevents smooth and gradual exhalation while breathing. (We colloquially refer to people being "too choked up" to speak.) He suggests that stuttering may occur when people force air through a constricted throat and across tense vocal cords as they speak. Helping stutterers control the airway dilation reflex that creates the problem is successful in reducing stuttering.

Other arousal-mediated responses, such as fidgeting, squirming, trembling, and so on, are presumably nothing more than overt manifestations of high internal arousal. When the sympathetic "fight or flight" reaction is activated by perceived threat, general arousal and muscular tension increase. This is appropriate preparation for fighting or fleeing from physical danger, but it is not a particularly adaptive response to social threats. Increased activation and tension beyond some optimal level does not help the speaker deliver a more effective address, extricate the highly embarrassed individual from his or her self-presentational predicament, or increase the likelihood that an adolescent will enjoy his or her date. In fact, high anxious arousal and its accompanying behaviors may actually interfere with facilitative social responses. Not only does the anxious individual behave more awkwardly and communicate less effectively, but arousal-mediated responses indicate to others that the person is nervous. In American culture, loss of poise is usually regarded negatively, so people try to conceal overt indices of their nervousness. Most of us have at one time or another attempted to control our jiggling feet, steady our shaking hands, force ourselves to breathe more slowly in an attempt to relax, or otherwise assume a countenance of poise and confidence when, in fact, we were actually very ill-at-ease.

Some behavioral manifestations of anxiety are more easily controlled than others. It is not too difficult to hold one's hands still by clasping them together or by grasping the podium, for example. It is a considerably greater feat to prevent them from perspiring! In addition, people seem to differ in the degree to which they are able to hide manifestations of their anxiety from others. Some people have acquired the knack of appearing poised and relaxed even when they are churning on the inside. They are seldom perceived as socially anxious or shy by others and may even be regarded as confident and extraverted (Leary & Schlenker, 1981; Zimbardo, 1977).

Other people are less fortunate, being less able to conceal their discomfort in social settings. Not being able to control behavioral manifestations of their inner arousal, such individuals may harbor even greater doubts that they will make the impressions they desire on others. In such cases, the social anxiety resulting from concerns with *appearing nervous* may be greater than the anxiety stemming from one's initial concerns with being evaluated unfavorably. I remember a student of mine who, when she became socially anxious, could not control her trembling hands, watering eyes, and the crimson splotches on her neck and face. I don't think she was more anxious than the average student when she was required to speak before the class, but her arousal-mediated responses were quite extreme. Upon talking to her privately, it was very clear that her social anxiety stemmed not from concerns with her ability to speak in front of the class per se but from the fear that she would tremble and turn red. The cycle was self-fulfilling as her worst fears came true each time she stood up to speak. Concerns about one's inability to control observable manifestations of anxiety can in themselves heighten anxiety and exacerbate arousal-mediated responses.

Since arousal-mediated responses may create additional difficulties for the highly socially anxious person, counselors and clinicians should inquire about the degree to which a socially anxious client is bothered by overt manifestations of his or her nervousness. If it appears that these sorts of responses are of concern, the client may be taught tactics for reducing the degree to which the nervousness is apparent. For example, keeping both feet on the floor prevents them from jiggling nervously. Breathing deeply and slowly helps the anxious individual to relax and control his or her quivering voice. Clasping one's hands together or grasping the podium will help to keep one's hands from trembling. These sorts of tactics should not be thought of as replacements for standard treatments of social anxiousness. Rather, they are of use as adjunct techniques for clients whose arousal-mediated responses heighten their interpersonal concerns. Of course, if the response in question is outside voluntary control (as in the case of the student whose face turns blotchy red), there is little that can be done superficially; treatment must focus directly on reduction of the anxiety itself.

Disaffiliation

Affiliation—seeking out and interacting with other people—is the most basic of all interpersonal processes. Without a desire to be with others, people would not have a social dimension to their lives at all and a great number of psychologists would have nothing to study. It is clear, however, that despite the gregariousness of human beings, certain psychological and social factors serve to reduce the amount of social contact people have with one another. Among the factors that reduce affiliation are many that are associated with social anxiety. People who feel socially anxious in an interpersonal encounter tend to *disaffiliate*—engage in actions that "serve to reduce the amount of social contact one individual has with another" (Leary, 1982, p. 111). When socially anxious, people tend to participate less fully in ongoing encounters, speak less to others, and often withdraw from anxiety-producing situations altogether.

The tendency for people to disaffiliate when socially anxious is particularly informative when it is compared to the findings of other research on affiliation. When people feel anxious for *nonsocial* reasons, such as an impending electric shock, the opposite effect—affiliation—is observed (Schachter, 1959). Taken together, these findings suggest that anxiety per se has no consistent effect upon affiliative behavior. Rather, affiliation is mediated by the cognitions people hold about the nature of the threat and the best way to deal with it. When anxiety arises for nonsocial reasons, people prefer to be with others—particularly with others who are facing a similar threat (Schachter, 1959). Affiliation under these circumstances is anxiety-reducing for many individuals (Wrightsman, 1960). However, in the case of social anxiety disaffiliation is preferred since the locus of the threat is other people. Being with others only heightens one's difficulties and discomfort. I will return to the nature of the relationship between social anxiety and disaffiliation in a few pages. But first, let us examine a few specific examples of the tendency for socially anxious people to disaffiliate.

REDUCED VERBAL BEHAVIOR

According to Zimbardo's (1977) surveys, most people say that the best indicator that people are feeling shy is that they do not talk very much. Of course, not everyone who is quiet in a social encounter is experiencing social anxiety; some people are simply more talkative than others. Nevertheless, numerous studies have shown that when people are socially anxious they are less likely to initiate conversations, they speak less often, talk a lower percentage of the time, take longer to respond to others, allow more silences to develop in conversations, and are less likely to break conversational silences once they occur (Arkowitz et al., 1975; Borkovec et al., 1974; Borkovec, Fleischmann, & Caputo, 1973; Cheek & Buss, 1981; Glasgow & Arkowitz, 1975; Leary, 1980, 1983b; Murray, 1971; Natale et al., 1979; Pilkonis, 1977b; Watson & Friend, 1969).[3]

It has also been found that situations in which people are reluctant to speak are characterized by factors that evoke concerns with others' evaluations. For example, people speak for a shorter length of time to critical, disapproving audiences and when addressing a large rather than a small audience (see Murray, 1971). People are also more reluctant to sing in front of those they believe are high in musical ability than in front of less talented audiences (Brown & Garland, 1972; Knight & Borden, 1978).

EYE CONTACT

Eye contact serves as an important channel of interpersonal communication. Since eye contact is associated with a desire to affiliate with others (Exline, Gray, & Schuette, 1965; Mehrabian, 1971), it is not surprising that when people are feeling socially anxious, they tend to look less at others and engage in less eye contact with them. Pilkonis (1977b) found that self-identified "shy" males look at others less than "nonshy" males, but obtained no difference in the gazing behavior of "shy" and "nonshy" females. Cheek and Buss (1981) found a nonsignificant tendency ($p<.15$) for shy women (identified by their Shyness Scale) to look at their conversation partner's face less than women who were lower in shyness. Situationally induced embarrassment—social anxiety caused by a specific self-presentational predicament—also results in decreased eye contact (Modigliani, 1971).

Gaze aversion seems to serve at least two functions for the socially anxious person. First, it helps shut out some of the threatening stimuli that are maintaining the anxiety and allows a degree of psychological withdrawal while one remains physically in the encounter. Although it stands as an untested proposition, it seems likely that gaze aversion actually reduces the intensity of the individual's social anxiety. Anxious individuals who are forced for reasons of decorum to maintain a high level of eye contact with the person who is the source of the anxiety should feel more anxious than those who are able to avert their gaze. Second, by failing to give others eye contact, the socially anxious interactant decreases the chances that others will initiate exchanges with him or her. People often wait until they have established eye contact before addressing another. By refusing to establish eye contact, the individual who wishes to disaffiliate discourages others from pulling him or her into conversations.

Although reduced eye contact may have advantages for the socially anxious person, it also has drawbacks. For instance, people like others more who give them a high degree of eye contact while interacting (LaFrance & Mayo, 1978). By failing to provide a high amount of eye contact, the socially anxious interactant may create a less favorable impression—the one thing he or she wishes most to avoid. Similarly, in public speaking situations, a high level of eye contact with members of the audience is associated with greater audience responsiveness. Also, people use low levels of eye contact as a clue that others are shy or socially anxious; reduced eye contact may advertise one's discomfort to others in the encounter (Zimbardo, 1977).

AVOIDANCE AND WITHDRAWAL

People may partially disaffiliate by reducing their eye contact and verbal participation in the encounter. Often, socially anxious people disaffiliate fully by actually leaving encounters in which they feel nervous or attempting to avoid them altogether (Twentyman & McFall, 1975; Watson & Friend, 1969; Zimbardo, 1977, 1981). As we saw earlier, people's scores on a number of measures of social anxiousness correlate negatively with extraversion and sociability (Cheek & Buss, 1981; Huntley, 1969; Leary, 1983a; Pilkonis, 1977a). Also, college students who score high on measures of shyness and social anxiousness date less frequently than students who score lower on these measures (Arkowitz et al., 1975; Glasgow & Arkowitz, 1975; Himadi, Arkowitz, Hinton, & Perl, 1980; Phibbs & Arkowitz, 1981; Twentyman & McFall, 1975).

McCroskey and Leppard (1975) found that college students who scored high on self-report measures of communication apprehension tended to choose living accommodations that were located such that they required less social interaction with others. Similarly, when in a small group setting, high communication apprehensives choose seating positions that require minimal interaction with other members of the group (Weiner, 1973). There is also data to suggest that socially anxious people interact with others at greater physical distances (Pilkonis, 1977b).

CAUSES OF DISAFFILIATION

Why do socially anxious people tend to disaffiliate by interacting less fully, giving others less eye contact, withdrawing prematurely from social encounters, and avoiding them altogether when possible? The answer to this question is not perfectly clear, probably because the relationship between anxiety and behavior is quite complex. What is clear is that disaffiliative responses do not appear to be *caused* by social anxiety, contrary to the commonsense notion that people do not interact fully *because* they are anxious. As I noted earlier in this chapter, when the source of one's anxiety is nonsocial, affiliation is increased rather than decreased. Anxiety itself does not automatically result in disaffiliation.

The disaffiliation that tends to accompany social anxiety appears to spring from at least three sources. First, social anxiety may serve as punishment for affiliative responses. Since anxiety is an inherently aversive experience, behaviors that are accompanied by anxiety are likely to decline in frequency while those that reduce social anxiety, such as disaffiliation, are likely to increase. In behavioristic terms, anxiety may be regarded as negative reinforcement for disaffiliative behaviors since an aversive stimulus (i.e., anxiety) is removed when the individual disaffiliates. It is not surprising that people will avoid those stimuli that produce aversive subjective reactions when possible.

A second way to view disaffiliation is by considering the plight of the socially anxious person. Given that the individual does not expect to receive the evaluations or reactions he or she desires, what purpose is there in staying in the encounter? When goal attainment (in this case, attaining social rewards) is judged impossible, the consequence (among other things) is withdrawal from future attempts to achieve the goal. (See Schlenker & Leary, 1982, for an application of Carver's, 1979, cybernetic model of self-attention to this point.) Put more simply, it is not worth the socially anxious person's effort to participate in social encounters in which no social rewards are anticipated.

Carrying this notion one step further suggests a third function of disaffiliation. Not only does the socially anxious individual not anticipate receiving social rewards, but the possibility remains that continued participation in the encounter will result in direct social costs. If I perceive that I am not coming across as well as I would like and feel helpless to improve my self-presentations to others, I may believe that my public image will be in jeopardy should I continue to participate in the encounter. Once I feel socially anxious, I am likely to think that things are only bound to get worse, so I withdraw. In the extreme case of embarrassment, in which the individual has clearly projected undesirable images, disaffiliation is often rapid and total, sometimes resulting in retreat from the encounter (Schlenker, 1980).

Consequences of Disaffiliative Tendencies

Luckily, occasional disaffiliation has few negative repercussions for people, particularly if one's withdrawal may be hidden behind the guise of other motives (e.g., "I hate to have to leave the party so early, but I have a lot of work to finish before tomorrow"). However, a chronic tendency to avoid or withdraw from social encounters may result in serious personal consequences for highly socially anxious individuals. I will discuss only four possible consequences.

LONELINESS

Nearly everyone experiences bouts of loneliness at times during their lives. A nationwide survey revealed that 26% of those contacted had felt "very lonely or remote from other people" during the preceding few weeks (Bradburn, 1969). Given their tendency to avoid social encounters and their difficulties initiating and maintaining conversations with others, it might be expected that people who are high in dispositional social anxiousness would be, on the average, more lonely than less socially anxious people.

In a study of the relationship between shyness and loneliness, Cheek & Busch (1981) used the Shyness Scale (Cheek & Buss, 1981) to classify college undergraduates into shy and nonshy groups. They then administered the revised UCLA Loneliness Scale

(Russell, Peplau, & Cutrona, 1980) during the first week of an academic semester and again two weeks before the end of the semester. (The Loneliness Scale is a 20-item self-report measure of the respondent's satisfaction-dissatisfaction with their current social relationships.) As expected, shy students reported being more lonely than nonshys both at the beginning and end of the semester.

In another study, Jones, Freemon, and Goswick (1981) showed that loneliness (as measured by the original UCLA Loneliness Scale) was significantly correlated with scores obtained on the social anxiety subscale of the Self-Consciousness Scale and the Social Reticence Scale. It has also been observed that people who are highly sensitive to rejection by others tend to be more lonely (Russell et al., 1980).

The most straightforward interpretation of this data is that highly socially anxious people tend to affiliate less, date less, and have fewer close friends, all of which results in greater loneliness. An alternative explanation is suggested by the fact that shy individuals tend to be regarded less positively by other people. Others find them generally less friendly and are less attracted to them (Jones & Russell, 1982). To the degree that this is true, highly shy or socially anxious people may be more lonely because others seek out their company less frequently.

The problem of loneliness is exacerbated by the fact that feelings of loneliness sensitize people to the evaluative aspects of interpersonal encounters (Peplau & Perlman, 1979). Because of their strong desire for social contact, lonely people tend to view others in terms of their potential for providing companionship, friendship, and romantic relationships. As a result, they approach social interactions highly motivated to get others to like and befriend them, and are highly attuned to others' reactions to them. This interpersonal orientation may heighten the social anxiety level of lonely people since they are both highly motivated to make particular impressions and are highly sensitive to the possibility of making negative impressions and being evaluated unfavorably. Heightened social anxiety may then be accompanied by further disaffiliation from potentially rewarding encounters and relationships, resulting in even greater loneliness. Such a spiraling cycle is difficult to break.

JOB PERFORMANCE AND SATISFACTION

Many occupations require employees to interact with other people or speak in front of groups on a regular basis. In other jobs, the interpersonal contact is minimal. The tendency to experience social anxiety and to wish to disaffiliate might have implications for the kinds of jobs people choose and for their performance and satisfaction in their jobs. There has been very little research on the occupational behavior of high and low socially anxious people, but the existing data are quite telling.

Daly and McCroskey (1975) found that subjects who scored high in communication apprehension—social anxiety experienced during oral communication—expressed a preference for occupations that require minimal oral communication. Subjects who were lower in communication apprehension desired to work in jobs that required a higher level of interpersonal communication. In addition, high communication apprehensives express greater dissatisfaction with jobs that require a high level of oral communication than low apprehensives (Falcione, McCroskey, & Daly, 1975).

In another study, McCroskey, Andersen, Richmond, and Wheeless (1981) surveyed 573 teachers in elementary and secondary schools. Teachers who scored high on the Personal Report of Communication Apprehension were overrepresented among teachers of grades 1 through 4. Apparently, highly socially anxious teachers are less troubled by dealing with younger children; research has shown that younger children are less likely to cause people to feel shy than are older children and adults (Zimbardo, 1977). Given the high interpersonal demands of teaching, future research is needed to examine the impact of social anxiousness on teachers' preferences, satisfaction, and teaching styles (McCroskey et al., 1981).

Similarly, industrial-organizational psychologists might do well to study the relationship between dispositional social anxiousness and satisfaction and performance in jobs that require a high level of interaction with others. Salespeople, flight attendants, social workers, personnel directors, teachers, and practicing psychologists are just a few of the professions that might be difficult and aversive for highly socially anxious individuals. Social anxiety would be expected to be less of a factor in more solitary occupations: assembly lines, truck driving, appliance repair, and so on. Along the same lines, measures of social anxiousness or the tendency to disaffiliate (i.e., a sociability scale) could conceivably be used to screen applicants for jobs requiring a high level of interpersonal contact.

Verbal participation in social encounters is often interpreted by others as a sign of leadership. That is, the selection of a person as leader of a small group is partly determined by the sheer quantity of the person's participation in the group (more so than the quality of what is said; Sorrentino & Boutillier, 1975). Inasmuch as this is the case, socially anxious people who disaffiliate may be less likely to be viewed as leaders, with obvious implications for job assignment and promotion to administrative positions. Indeed, socially anxious and shy individuals are less likely than other people to be perceived as possessing leadership capabilities (Jones & Russell, 1982; McCroskey, 1975). In an extensive study of cadets at West Point, Zimbardo and his colleagues (reported in Zimbardo, 1980) examined the relationship between shyness and cadets' "leadership effectiveness scores"—a composite of several judges' ratings of their leadership capability. Shy cadets had leadership effectiveness scores that were significantly lower than less shy cadets. In a related vein, research by Harrell (reported in Zimbardo, 1980) showed that the best predictors of success in business are sociability and verbal fluency. Since socially anxious people tend to be less sociable, less talkative, and less fluent, they may tend to be less successful in business ventures. In sum, the tendency for socially anxious people to disaffiliate has serious consequences for job preference, satisfaction, and performance, consequences that deserve a great deal more research attention.

SEXUAL BEHAVIOR

Interactions with persons of the other sex are highly anxiety-arousing for a high proportion of the population, particularly for those in adolescence and young adulthood (e.g., Arkowitz et al., 1978; Glass et al., 1976; Martinson & Zerface, 1970; Zimbardo, 1977, 1981). Since episodes of social anxiety are often accompanied by disaffiliation, it is not surprising that individuals who score high on self-report measures of social anxiousness report that they date less frequently and have fewer interpersonal contacts with those of the other sex than less socially anxious individuals (Himadi et al., 1980; Twentyman & McFall, 1975). Taking the developmental progression of interpersonal dealings one step further, it is also likely that socially anxious people become involved in fewer casual and long-term heterosexual relationships, thereby limiting the availability of satisfying sexual experiences.

Not only does social avoidance limit one's interpersonal contacts with the other sex, but sexual encounters themselves are characterized by a number of factors that we have already seen exacerbate social anxiety and disaffiliation. Sexual encounters are often highly ambiguous (i.e., there are no hard and fast rules to guide one's behavior), engender a high fear of being evaluated negatively for one's appearance or sexual performance, induce a high level of public self-awareness, and present possible risks to central aspects of one's self-concept. These factors seem to make it less likely that people who experience high social anxiety in mundane encounters will initiate or respond to sexual overtures.

To examine the relationship between social anxiety and sexual behavior, Leary and Dobbins (1983) conducted a comprehensive study of the sexual experiences of 260 unmarried college undergraduates. Using a modification of the Survey of Heterosexual Interactions as a measure of respondents' levels of heterosocial anxiousness (defined as the tendency to experience social anxiety in real, anticipated, or imagined interactions with those of the other sex), they found that social anxiety experienced in mundane heterosocial interactions was strongly related to respondents' sexual experiences.

First, a lower percentage of highly socially anxious subjects reported that they had engaged in sexual intercourse. Of the low heterosocially anxious males, 84% reported that they had had sex, compared to 71% of the high anxious males; 68% of the low and 57% of the high socially anxious females reported having experienced intercourse. As would be expected, highly socially anxious subjects reported a lower frequency of intercourse in the past month and a smaller number of sexual partners than less socially anxious students. Also, highly socially anxious women were less likely to have engaged in oral sex than less anxious women; the difference for men was also in the expected direction, although only marginally significant. Zimbardo (1977) also reports differences in intercourse, petting, and oral sex between "shy" and "nonshy" respondents as identified by the single self-report item on the Shyness Survey. Taken together, these findings portray the socially anxious student as less sexually experienced than less anxious students.

Social anxiousness was related to contraceptive use among women but not among men. Although high and low socially anxious women used some form of contraception equally often, there were pronounced differences in the types of birth control used. Low socially anxious women were much more likely to be on the pill while a higher percentage of high than low socially anxious women indicated that their partner had used a condom the last time they had had sex. It appears that low heterosocially anxious women were more likely to use modes of contraception that required preplanning on their part (e.g., pill and diaphragm) than highly anxious women.

In some ways, this finding is surprising if one assumes (as we did) that the "negotiation" required when the couple uses a condom would be particularly embarrassing for women who scored high in heterosocial anxiousness. Two possible explanations come to mind. First, since the pill tends to be used by more sexually active women and the low socially anxious women were more sexually active, their prefernce for the pill may reflect their higher expectancy of having sex. Women who were more socially anxious (and less sexually active) may have felt less need to take the pill. A second possibility is that highly socially anxious women are deterred from using the pill (and diaphragm) because they find the prospect of going to a physician for contraception highly anxiety-evoking. They choose to deal with birth control at the time of each sexual encounter rather than go through (what may be to them) the traumatic experience of seeking contraception themselves.[4]

The sexual lives of highly socially anxious people may also be adversely affected by anxious arousal itself. A high proportion of cases of sexual disfunction, such as premature ejaculation and failure to reach orgasm, are brought about by a high level of anxiety (Hyde, 1982). Leary and Dobbins (in press) found that a somewhat higher proportion of high than low socially anxious men reported having experienced temporary impotence and premature ejaculation. Also, a lower proportion of high than low socially anxious women said that they had ever had an orgasm. Sexually active respondents who were high in social anxiousness also indicated that they had enjoyed their recent sexual encounters less than those low in social anxiousness.

In sum, a high level of dispositional social anxiousness regarding cross-sex encounters is related to less sexual experience, specific patterns of contraceptive use, and a higher level of sexual difficulties. Clinicians and counselors should be attuned to the possibility that clients' sexual complaints may be related to a high degree of social anxiousness and the accompanying tendency to disaffiliate (see Solomon & Solomon, 1971; Zimbardo, 1977).

ALCOHOL DEPENDENCE

Alcohol dependence may serve any of several social and psychological needs for the problem drinker. One such function is to cope with frustration, anxiety, and feelings of personal inadequacy. Given the picture we have painted of the extremely socially anxious individual—inhibited, lonely, anxious, fearful of negative evaluations—we might hypothesize that a higher percentage of high than low socially anxious people are alcoholics. People may begin to drink in order to relax in anxiety-producing social situations (Zimbardo, 1977).

To cite an anecdotal example, country singer Kris Kristofferson who battled alcohol for several years notes that, "Ever since I started performing, I've had these anxiety attacks about going on stage. I'd even get nervous the night before, I needed the courage to perform, and I found it by drinking" (*Columbus Dispatch,* 1981).

In addition to reducing social anxiety, alcohol use may serve as a self-handicapping strategy (Jones & Berglas, 1978). When people are afraid of the personal implications of failure, they may use alcohol so that their social failures may be attributed to the alcohol rather than to their personal inadequacies.

Hull, Young, and Swank (1981) administered the Self-Consciousness Scale (Fenigstein et al., 1975) to 35 male alcoholics who were completing an alcohol detoxification program at a V.A. hospital. They then assessed the proportion of high versus low socially anxious subjects who had relapsed to a pretreatment level of alcohol use at three and six months after the conclusion of the detox program. After three months, over three times as many high as low socially anxious subjects had relapsed (67% versus 18%). At the end of six months, 78% of the highs, compared to 41% of the lows had relapsed. In a study of 178 college students, Maroldo (1983) found that alcohol consumption correlated positively with scores on a measure of shyness, although only for male respondents. Although more research is needed to fully understand the link between social concerns and alcohol use (see Hull, Levenson, Young, & Sher, 1983, for one approach), it is clear that social anxiousness is implicated in alcohol abuse. Given the importance of this area, it obviously deserves more research attention.

Self-Presentation

We have examined two of the three categories of behavioral concomitants of social anxiety: arousal-mediated responses and disaffiliation. I will conclude this chapter with a look at the third category—those behaviors of socially anxious people that appear to serve self-presentational functions.

Consider for a moment the plight of the person who feels nervous in an interpersonal encounter. According to the self-presentation theory, he or she is motivated to make certain kinds of impressions upon other interactants, but believes he or she will be unsuccessful at doing so. If the situation is sufficiently aversive and withdrawal from the encounter is possible, the anxious individual may choose to leave the situation entirely. If this can be accomplished without a loss of face, the person's self-presentational problems are over, at least for the present. But what of the individual who is experiencing a great deal of distress but *cannot* withdraw?

We have already seen that the individual may attempt to partially disaffiliate by talking less, reducing eye contact, and so on. In addition, I would expect such individuals to try to enhance and/or protect their self-presentations as best they can under the circumstances. Although they do not think they will be able to make the kinds of impressions they would like to make, they would still want to maintain as appropriate a social image as possible (Leary & Schlenker, 1981; Zimbardo, 1981). They are not coming across as well as they would like, and feel nervous as the result, but they will want to be sure they do not come across *badly*.

Zimbardo (1981) suggests that, when socially anxious, people are likely to adopt a "protective" as opposed to an "acquisitive" self-presentation style. Arkin (1981) distinguishes between these two basic modes of self-presentation by noting that protective self-presentations involve attempts to avoid losses in social approval and/or attempts to avoid disapproval, whereas acquisitive self-presentations aim to gain social approval. In other words, we might expect socially anxious people's self-presentational attempts to be confined to relatively safe bets. They will want to convey self-images that carry little risk and will want to avoid jeopardizing their images if they can help it. They are unlikely to attempt to portray highly attractive images or make exaggerated claims that they may have difficulty sustaining. It is safer to employ subtle, low-risk strategies. Only one study has been conducted to examine the self-presentations of highly socially anxious people (Leary, 1983b). However, several studies shed some indirect light on this topic.

INNOCUOUS SOCIABILITY

What types of impressions might an individual attempt to foster that convey desired attributes yet carry little social risk? First, there is some evidence that, when people feel socially anxious, they attempt to appear—for lack of a better term—innocuously sociable (Leary, 1982; Schlenker & Leary, 1982). For example, they are likely to behave in ways that indicate interest in and agreement with what others are saying. Women who are shy smile more frequently during conversations and nod their heads (as if agreeing) more often. As Pilkonis (1977b, p. 603) observes, "it appears that shy females, anxious to make a good impression but constrained by a somewhat limited role, are able to achieve their goal through frequent nodding and smiling."

Natale et al. (1979) found that subjects who scored high on the Social Avoidance and Distress Scale interrupted others less often, yet were more likely to use back-channel responses—those sounds that a listener makes to indicate that he or she is attentive to another (such as "uh-huh"). Such responses serve to convey an image of friendliness, politeness, interest, and agreeableness, while allowing the anxious interactant to be minimally involved in the encounter. Attentive listeners win friends; I have heard people remark of a shy friend, "He's awfully quiet, but he seems like a nice guy."

Since low-risk self-presentations of innocuous sociability have interpersonal benefits for the individual, counselors and clinicians might suggest that highly socially anxious clients adopt these sorts of responses in those instances in which they feel incapable of participating fully in social encounters.

Such behaviors serve not only to project mildly positive images of the person but also help keep the anxious individual out of the social spotlight. Smiling, nodding, and attentiveness prompt other interactants to dominate the conversation. Although having someone else monopolize the conversation is irritating to many people, it is a blessing for the socially anxious person who prefers to remain silent. An interesting hypothesis is that a higher percentage of socially anxious people's contributions to conversations are in the form of questions. Asking other interactants about themselves allows the anxious person to appear interested in others, reduces the need to talk about him- or herself, prompts others to dominate the conversation, and keeps his or her own contributions safe and minimal (Efran & Korn, 1969).

Carried to an extreme, what I have been calling innocuous sociability may involve a full lack of assertiveness which in fact may be quite nocuous to others. Afraid of saying or doing something others might view negatively, people may refuse to express themselves openly when appropriate and may even appear to be *too* sociable and agreeable. A letter to "Dear Abby" illustrated this point. It was from a woman who was frustrated with a freidn's extreme passivity. This friend would never give a direct answer to even such a simple question as whether or not she would like a cup of coffee. When finally pressed to make a definite statement, she realized how annoying her lack of assertiveness had been to others. It was the result, she admitted, of being shy and afraid that others might not accept her if she came across as too forward or eager. As this letter shows, total passivity may seem safe but may actually be a social hindrance. In counseling socially anxious people it may be necessary to stress the value of being positive and assertive.

IMPRESSIONS OF SIMILARITY

People like those whom they perceive to be similar to themselves (Byrne, 1971). For example, as the proportion of similar attitudes that two people hold in common increases, their liking for one another increases in a linear fashion (Byrne & Nelson, 1965). People also rate similar others as more knowledgeable, intelligent, and adjusted than dissimilar others (Byrne, 1971). After all, who would say that similar others are maladjusted nincompoops?

Armed with the intuitive knowledge that perceived similarity increases attraction, people attempt to convey the impression of being similar to those they are motivated to impress (Davis & Florquist, 1965; Jellison & Gentry, 1978; Jones, Gergen, Gumpert, & Thibaut, 1965; Jones, Gergen, & Jones, 1963). In cases in which the individual is truly similar to another, he or she will simply want to make that fact known. In other instances, people feign similarity to enhance another's liking for them. By overplaying areas of agreement, people increase their chances of being evaluated positively by others and reduce the likelihood of criticism and rejection.

The tactic of emphasizing one's similarity to another may be particularly useful to people who are experiencing social anxiety since, if used discretely, it entails little risk. (The risk comes from the target's possible suspicion that the person really doesn't agree with him or her.) Although little research has been conducted to examine the ingratiation attempts of socially anxious people, one study showed the expected pattern (Turner, 1977). In this study, subjects classified as dispositionally high or low in social anxiousness were told that they would hear a tape of an expert arguing against a position the subjects believed in (that a cure for cancer was soon coming). Prior to actually hearing the tape, subjects' beliefs about the possibility of finding a cure for cancer were reassessed. Subjects high in social anxiousness showed a shift in their beliefs toward the position advocated by the expert, whereas low anxious subjects did not. By adopting a more moderate position, highly socially anxious subjects were able to increase their perceived similarity with the expert, reduce the possibility of argument with others about a cure for cancer, and, ultimately, forestall the possibility of being evaluated negatively for holding a "wrong" or indefensible belief. Other research has shown that people demonstrate "anticipatory attitude change" as a self-presentational tactic in such situations (e.g., Hass & Mann, 1976) but the role of social anxiety in the effect has not been adequately assessed.

Related to managing the impression of similarity is conformity. Since people who conform to others' opinions and to group norms are better liked, we might expect socially anxious people to be more conforming. Indeed, Zimbardo (1980) presents evidence that people who are shy are more conforming and more easily persuaded than less shy people.

PROSOCIAL BEHAVIOR

Another way to project favorable impressions of oneself to others is to be seen doing helpful and thoughtful sorts of things for people. Thus, we might expect that socially anxious people go out of their way to do nice things in order to be evaluated positively. However, helping and favor-doing often carry a degree of social risk. It is often difficult, for example, to determine when helping is appropriate. It is clearly proper to help an elderly man pick up the packages he dropped in the store, but should you offer to get the attractive man or woman at the party another drink? Will he or she think you are too forward? Will he/she thank you coldly, then get the drink him- or herself? Will your friends kid you for appearing to "come on" to this person? Will you mix the drink properly? These are the kinds of questions that buzz in the heads of socially anxious people when they contemplate doing a favor for another.

But what about when help is more clearly needed, such as in an emergency? Wouldn't the socially anxious person be first in line to help so as to make a good impression? Based upon the research on prosocial behavior in social psychology, the answer is "probably not." A primary cause of people's failures to help in emergency situations is a concern with looking foolish or being evaluated negatively (Latane & Darley, 1970). Being helpful, even in an emergency, puts the helper's behavior, characteristics, and motives under others' scrutiny, and raises the possibility that the proffered help was inappropriate or that the individual will botch up the attempt in front of the victim and onlookers. As a result, it appears that people who are high in social anxiousness are *less* likely to engage in prosocial behavior than those low in social anxiousness and this is particularly true when they must break a social norm in order to help (McGovern, 1976). The potential image-enhancement associated with helping is not worth the risk.

What about when people are explicitly asked for help? In such cases, socially anxious people should be more likely to help since failure to do so might be regarded negatively by others. People who are embarrassed by acting foolishly in front of others are more likely to comply with others' requests for assistance than those who are not embarrassed. In some studies, subjects have been led to perform behaviors that made them look ridiculous to other subjects, such as dancing wildly to a disco record, singing "The Star Spangled Banner" *a cappella,* or pretending to throw a temper tantrum. Afterwards, subjects were asked by another student to volunteer to help on a class project by filling out a questionnaire for 30 minutes a day for a month (no small request). Compared to subjects who did not perform embarrassing behaviors, embarrassed subjects agreed to complete the questionnaire for a greater number of days (Apsler, 1975; Miller, 1979).

Whether people who are experiencing social anxiety for other reasons, such as having to give a speech, are also more likely to comply with requests for help has not been investigated. I would guess that they would be. Social anxiety appears to increase prosocial behavior when help is explicitly requested but decrease helping when it is not.

SELF-DESCRIPTIONS

The most direct way of presenting particular images of oneself to others is through self-descriptions, the written and spoken expressions of information about oneself (Schlenker, 1980). How might the self-descriptions of interactants be affected by the factors that heighten social anxiety? Although it might seem that socially anxious people would try to present highly attractive images of themselves in order to be evaluated as they desire, we must remember that, when socially anxious, people doubt that they will make the kinds of impressions they wish to. Their low self-presentational efficacy constrains the positivity of their self-descriptions. Under normal circumstances, highly socially anxious people should be more self-effacing than less anxious individuals.

However, under other circumstances, situational factors may ease the perceived constraints on socially anxious people's self-presentations. This point is nicely demonstrated in an experiment I recently completed (Leary, 1983b). After subjects reported to the laboratory in opposite-sexed pairs, they completed the Interaction Anxiousness Scale (Leary, 1983a) and were classified as either low or high in dispositional social anxiousness. They were then told that the study was designed to investigate the effects of background noise on interpersonal behavior. They were to have a conversation to get to know one another while tape-recorded "party" noise was played into the room. Half of the subjects were told that they were in the "loud noise" condition; they were led to believe that we expected the noise to be quite disruptive and annoying, and that they would have some difficulty communicating and getting to know one another. The other half of the subjects were told they were in the "soft noise" condition and that the effects of the noise on their ability to converse with one another would be minimal. In fact, all subjects heard the noise tape at the same loudness (moderately loud). After their five-minute conversation, subjects completed (among other measures) a self-descriptive questionnaire that they believed would be seen by the other subject. Since their self-descriptions would be public, their responses on the questionnaire could be regarded as a measure of their self-presentations to the other subject.

Before describing the results, let us consider the experimental setting from the socially anxious subject's vantage point. What effect should the supposed loudness of the noise have on their self-presentations after the conversation? In the so-called "soft noise" condition (remember that the actual loudness of the noise was held constant) subjects should assume that their conversation partners had formed a clear-cut impression of them. There was no reason for anyone to assume that the subject was in any way different from the way he or she was perceived to be during the conversation. In this case, self-presentations after the conversation must be consistent with how the subject believed he or she was perceived by the other person; overly positive self-descriptions would be rejected. Since, all other things being equal, highly socially anxious people doubt that they can make highly favorable impressions on others, their self-descriptions should be less positive than those of subjects low in social anxiousness but only in the "soft noise" condition.

In the "loud noise" condition, subjects who thought the noise was supposed to be loud and disruptive might think that their conversation partner had not formed a confident impression of them. After all, the experimenter had said that they would have difficulty getting to know one another. With the "loud" noise as an external impediment, the subject's behavior during the conversation cannot be taken as a direct reflection of her or her personal characteristics. In attribution terms, subjects should assume that "discounting" will occur. As a result, the socially anxious subjects' postexperimental self-presentations are not constrained by how they behaved during the conversation itself.

The results clearly supported this line of reasoning. When subjects thought the noise was to be soft and nondisruptive, highly socially anxious subjects' self-descriptions were significantly less positive than those of less anxious subjects. However, in the "loud" noise condition, high and low socially anxious subjects described themselves equally positively on the self-presentation questionnaire. What this suggests is that, under normal circumstances, highly socially anxious people do not try to present as positive a social image of themselves as lows. However, when situational factors appear to prevent others from independently forming confident impressions of them, highly socially anxious people describe themselves as positively as low socially anxious people.[5]

DISCLAIMERS AND ACCOUNTS

People who are feeling socially anxious are worried that others will interpret their actions in ways that reflect badly upon them. To prevent this, they may use verbal statements that attempt to lead others to draw the "best" conclusions about them.

Disclaimers are statements people make in advance of performing actions that others might interpret negatively to dispel any unfavorable impressions that might be created (Hewitt &

Stokes, 1975). As such, they should be used more often by people who are apprehensive about others' evaluations of them. For example, a socially anxious person might hedge his or her statements with phrases such as "I might be wrong, but it seems to me that..." or "I haven't really thought this through, but..." Such phrases show others that the individual has no misconceptions that what he or she is saying is perfectly accurate or sensible. If others react critically to what is said, the person can respond, "As I said, it was just a thought," allowing him or her to avoid negative reactions. Through disclaimers, people reduce some of the self-presentational risks that accompany all interactions. The hypothesis that the use of disclaimers increases during episodes of social anxiety and is greater among high than low dispositionally socially anxious people awaits empirical attention.

Disclaimers are used *in advance* of potentially image-threatening events to ward off negative evaluations and reactions from others. Accounts, on the other hand, are explanations used *after* an event has occurred that has cast the individual in an unfavorable light (Schlenker, 1980). For example, people may use excuses to minimize their apparent responsibility for the undesirable event or justifications to reduce the perceived undesirability of the event itself. In either case, if the individual believes that his or her accounts have been accepted by others and his or her social image has been repaired, feelings of social anxiety should abate.

Summary

The behaviors that accompany episodes of social anxiety may be classified into three general categories. Arousal-mediated responses include those behaviors that are more or less directly affected by arousal of the sympathetic nervous system, such as fidgeting, stammering, and trembling. Socially anxious people also tend to disaffiliate (reduce their social contact with others) by talking less, reducing eye contact, withdrawing from encounters in which they feel nervous, and often avoiding them entirely. The tendency to disaffiliate has a number of consequences for highly socially anxious people. They tend to be more lonely, are more dissatisfied with jobs that require a high degree of interpersonal contact, have more limited sexual experiences but greater sexual difficulties, and may become dependent upon alcohol in order to reduce their social insecurities. Finally, when socially anxious, people engage in self-presentational behaviors in an attempt to project as favorable an image as possible in anxiety-producing social settings.

Notes

1. I am purposefully using the phrase "behavioral concomitants" rather than "behavioral effects" because, as will become clear below, many of the behaviors that accompany episodes of social anxiety are not, in fact, *caused* by anxiety. Rather, they are the effects of the same kinds of factors that precipitate anxiety itself.
2. The literatures on test anxiety and social anxiety are intimately related since they both deal with concerns about being evaluated. An integrative review of the two areas is badly needed since researchers in each area have much to gain from those in the other. I would like to proffer one idea regarding test anxiety. It seems that some sources of test anxiety are social in nature, arising from the prospect or presence of interpersonal evaluation ("My parents will be mad if I fail this test"), whereas other sources of test anxiety are nonsocial ("If I don't do well on this test, I won't get the job, and the bank will foreclose on my house"). In studying and treating test anxiety, this distinction may be of use.
3. One must be careful when interpreting some of the research dealing with "shyness" and disaffiliation. Since some measures of shyness assess inhibited and avoidant behavior in addition to social anxiousness, studies that use such measures say little about the link between social anxiety and disaffiliation directly. Rather, they demonstrate specific manifestations of "shy" behavior.
4. I am indebted to Barry Schlenker for this alternative explanation.
5. In addition to resulting in more positive self-presentations, the so-called loud noise condition also lowered the arousal level of dispositionally socially anxious subjects (as measured by pulse rates). Apparently, believing that the other person would have difficulty forming confident impressions of them in the loud noise condition reduced anxious subjects' self-presentational concerns and lowered social anxiety.

7

THE DEVELOPMENT OF INDIVIDUAL DIFFERENCES

Individuals differ widely in the frequency and intensity with which they experience social anxiety across different situations and over time. It is easy for us to categorize those we know (and ourselves, for that matter) along a continuum of social anxiousness. At one end are those people who are typically relaxed, confident, and poised in most social encounters, while at the other are those who are nervous and unsure of themselves a high percentage of the time. How might these differences among individuals be explained? In this chapter, we will examine this important question.

Individual Differences

For clarification, let us first consider what is meant when we refer to social anxiousness as an *individual difference* variable. Terms that allude to psychological characteristics, (such as trait, disposition, and personality) have had a checkered past in psychology. In fact, many contemporary psychologists hesitate to use such constructs. Some of the objections have arisen in response to early trait theorists who assumed that psychic or neurological structures of some sort underlie all traits (Hogan, DeSoto, & Solano, 1977). Most modern personality researchers make no such assumptions. Instead, traits or dispositions are defined as observed stylistic consistencies or regularities in people's behavior, affect, or cognition. Since the existence of a trait assumes differences among individuals on that trait, such constructs are commonly referred to as individual difference variables. For many, the term "individual difference" is more palatable than "trait" or "personality characteristic" since it is simply a descriptive term and carries none of the historical connotations of the other terms. For our purposes, social anxiousness may just as easily be called a trait, a disposition, a personality characteristic, or an individual difference variable. Whatever it is called, we simply mean that individuals demonstrate a degree of cross-situational consistency in their tendency to experience social anxiety, and differ among themselves in the frequency and intensity with which they do so (see Cattell, 1973; Comrey, 1965; Crozier, 1979).

For reasons that will become apparent below, I would like to suggest that social anxiousness is best regarded as (for lack of a better term) a second-order individual difference variable. By this, I mean that individual differences in social anxiousness appear to occur because of individual differences in several other, more basic psychological characteristics. Although social anxiousness is a meaningful dimension upon which people may be classified, individual differences in social anxiousness are reducible to other characteristics.

This will become clearer if we modify the central proposition of the self-presentation theory of social anxiety so that it accounts for individual differences in social anxiousness. The self-presentation approach suggests that people differ in *dispositional* social anxiousness to the degree that they differ on other personality characteristics that are associated with (you guessed it) the motivation to make particular impressions upon others or the tendency to doubt that one will make desired impressions. People who possess characteristics that predispose them to desire to make impressions on others or hold a low self-presentational efficacy will experience social anxiety more often than people who do not possess such characteristics. Put another way, they will be high in social anxiousness.

Note that dispositional social anxiousness will be heightened by possessing characteristics related to *either* of the factors that precipitate social anxiety; both sets of factors are not needed to predispose a person to be high in social anxiousness. (Both factors *are* necessary to actually experience the state of social anxiety.) Before focusing directly on personality characteristics that may underlie social anxiousness, let us speculate regarding the role of temperamental factors.

Temperament and Social Anxiety

Interest in temperamental factors and their relationship to social behavior has grown substantially in recent years. A temperament is a broad, inherited personality disposition (Allport, 1961). It refers to observed consistencies in styles of behavior or affect that are unlearned and for which there is evidence of a genetic component (Buss & Plomin, 1975). Of course, strictly speaking, neither behavior, cognition, nor affect are inhereited directly from one's parents. Rather, what may be inherited is a nervous system that is structured in such a fashion that certain kinds of responses occur more easily and frequently than others. The existence of a temperament does not imply that the person's responses may not be modified by environmental factors, only that he or she has inherited a physical constitution that affects behavior in specific, consistent ways.

Is there any evidence that social anxiousness has an inherited component? Although social anxiousness measured independently of social behavior has not been directly studied, there are informative data on related constructs. Among his 16 personality factors, Cattell (1973) identified a dimension that he called the "H-negative" or "threctic" personality. Threctic people tend to be shy, timid, restrained, and overly sensitive to physical *and social* threats. They are contrasted with paramic individuals who are adventurous, confident in interpersonal encounters, and "thick-skinned." His data show that threctia has an inherited component; the heritability coefficient (h^2) is .40. (Heritability is the proportion of variance in an observed characteristic that is accounted for by genetic factors.) Cattell hypothesized that threctics are highly responsive to threatening situations because their sympathetic nervous systems have a low threshold for activation.

More recently, Cheek and Zonderman (presented in Cheek, 1982) administered the Cheek and Buss (1981) Shyness Scale to 839 pairs of monozygotic (identical) and dizygotic (fraternal) twins. As would be expected if a genetic component were involved in shyness, the correlation between the shyness scores for monozygotic twins was significantly greater than the correlation for dizygotic twins.[1] Based on their data, heritability estimates of .68 for males and .50 for females were calculated.

It seems likely that the genetic underpinnings of shyness and social anxiousness lie in emotionality, one of the four basic temperaments identified by Buss and Plomin (1975). Emotionality refers to temperamental differences in how intensely people respond to stimuli, differences that are easily observable in neonates. Some individuals—those who are high in emotionality—are more easily aroused by stimuli of all sorts and experience their emotions more deeply. Buss and Plomin (1975) report a large body of data that support the notion that individual differences in emotionality are partially due to temperamental factors. Although the anatomical and physiological substrates of temperamental emotionality have not been identified, it is reasonable to assume, as Cattell (1973) did, that some individuals' nervous systems are more arousable than others and these individuals thus experience all emotions, including social anxiety, more often than other individuals.

Berberian and Snyder (1982) conducted a study of infants that lends support to the hypothesized link between temperamental emotionality and anxiousness. Taking measures of temperament from 60 infants, they then observed their reactions to the approach of a stranger. Correlational data showed that infants who were temperamentally fussy and difficult tended to be more fearful and less friendly when approached by the stranger than did the temperamentally "easy-going" infants. Similarly, Scarr and Salapatek (1970) found that fearfulness to a stranger was associated with general negativity, nonadaptivity, avoidance of new situations and a low sensory threshold. Apparently, inherited predispositions toward arousability and emotionality may account for some individual differences in social anxiousness. A great deal more research is needed on this question, however.

Developmental Antecedents

Although temperamental variables may account for some of the variability among individuals in social anxiousness, there is no doubt that experience plays a large role. As I mentioned earlier, individual differences in social anxiousness may be traced to differences in other, more basic personality attributes—attributes that are strongly affected by experience and learning. To fully explore the development of the characteristics that seem to underlie dispositional social anxiousness would require a great deal more space than this chapter permits. Therefore, I will focus primarily on only four such characteristics. Two of these may be hypothesized to underlie social anxiousness because they are associated with a high level of motivation to make particular impressions on others (public self-consciousness and need for approval). The other two are related to social anxiousness because they are associated with a low sense of self-presentational efficacy (self-esteem and social skills).

PUBLIC SELF-CONSCIOUSNESS

We saw in Chapter 4 that an awareness of oneself as the object of others' scrutiny is a necessary condition for the experience of social anxiety (Buss, 1980). People will not be motivated to manage their impressions unless they are aware that they are being perceived and evaluated by others. It is clear, then, that children will not feel socially anxious until they have developed the capacity to be consciously aware of themselves and to be concerned with how they are evaluated by other people. Many parents may object to this assertion, insisting that their children showed signs of being anxious in social settings long before the child was able to think about himself or herself objectively. Even very young babies become distressed in the presence of strangers and in novel social encounters. As early as the seventh month of life, babies cry, show increased heartrate, and attempt to withdraw when strangers are present (Stroufe, 1977). Among preschoolers, strangers are more likely to induce shylike behavior than any other factor (Zimbardo, 1977, 1981). Is this not evidence of social anxiety in the absence of public self-awareness?

The reactions observed in babies and young children, properly designated *stranger anxiety* or *wariness,* are not evidence of preconscious social anxiety. Although these responses may occur in reaction to social factors, they are more akin to fears of unknown objects than to social anxiety. Very young children are often fearful of a variety of novel stimuli, including unfamiliar animals, strange sounds, new toys (such as puppets and masks), and unknown people. The cause of wariness in young children is the presence of unfamiliar or threatening stimuli, not the prospect or presence of interpersonal evaluation as is the case in social anxiety (see Greenberg & Marvin, 1982).

As Mead (1934), Cooley (1922), and others have observed, the ability to take the perspectives of others vis-à-vis oneself is necessary for most adult social behavior, including, I may add, the "ability" to experience social anxiety. The capacity to take the viewpoint of others when thinking about oneself does not generally emerge until age 4 or 5. Thus, we would not expect to observe true social anxiety until around that age.

Once people have developed the ability to view themselves as an object, they are able to contemplate how they are perceived and evaluated by others. As we saw in Chapter 4, however, individuals differ in their tendency to think about the public aspects of themselves (Buss, 1980; Fenigstein et al., 1975). People who are *high* in public self-consciousness think about how they are coming across to others a great deal of the time and are more sensitive to others' implicit and explicit evaluations of them (Fenigstein, 1979). People who are *low* in public self-consciousness are less aware of and, apparently, less interested in how they are perceived and regarded by others. Since publicly self-conscious people are more likely to be high in dispositional social anxiousness (Fenigstein et al., 1975; Leary, 1983a), it is of interest to speculate regarding the developmental antecedents of public self-consciousness.

Children of highly publicly self-conscious parents may learn to be publicly self-conscious through modeling processes. Children who observe that mom and dad are very concerned with how they (the parents) are evaluated by others are likely to learn to adopt greater self-scrutiny than children of parents who are not obviously concerned with others' evaluations. One can imagine a child witnessing and then internalizing parents' expressed concerns about social evaluation. When parents often express concerns with what neighbors, friends, family, and coworkers think about the appearance of the family car, the parents' clothing, an infraction by one of their children, or the prestige of the parents' occupations, children may come to believe that it is important to consider others' perceptions and evaluations of oneself.

At the same time, highly self-conscious parents may directly admonish their children to behave in ways that will make the "right" impressions: "What will the neighbors think if they see you... screaming like this/sitting in the car for too long with your date/coming in at all hours of the night/drinking beer/etc?" Parents may convey to their children that the standards for judging the appropriateness of behavior are others' reactions to it. An emphasis on the child's appearance and clothing should also help foster public self-consciousness: "You can't go out dressed like that—people will think you're a slob/tramp/orphan/etc."

After completing the Self-Consciousness Scale and learning that she scored very high in public self-consciousness, a student of mine shared with me what she saw as the cause of her overconcern with others' perceptions of her. Her parents were, by most people's standards, loving, dedicated, and concerned. However, they often expressed a great deal of apprehension about how other people viewed them and their children. Interested in assuring that their children were dressed nicely, the parents insisted on the children wearing perfectly matched, coordinated outfits to school every day. The children were regularly prompted to think about how their actions were seen by others and were instructed to always behave in ways that other people would deem acceptable. The parents seemed to be particularly concerned about what their friends thought of their children. When my student gained weight during her freshman year at college, her parents reacted as if it were, in her words, "the worst tragedy that ever hit our family." They expressed embarrassment at being seen with her, although, aside from a few extra pounds, she was an attractive woman. They also went overboard in an attempt to help her with her "problem," including sending her to a physician, a nutritionist, and a psychologist. Throughout all of this, their emphasis was clearly on helping their daughter *look better,* not on reducing her weight for health reasons. Given her parents' overattention to their and their children's public selves, it is not at all surprising that my student scored two standard deviations above the mean on the Public Self-Consciousness Scale.

A concern for how one is viewed by others has been implicated in a number of interpersonal phenomena, including conformity, self-presentation, socialization, self-serving attributions, and, of course, social anxiety. Clearly, a great deal more research attention should be directed toward the developmental antecedents of public self-consciousness (see, Buss, 1980, for other thoughts on this topic). In addition, research is needed to examine ways of reducing chronically high levels of self-consciousness. Treatments that focus on public self-consciousness might be quite useful for a certain subset of socially anxious clients.

NEED FOR APPROVAL

People who are highly motivated to obtain social approval and avoid disapproval seem to be predisposed to experience social anxiety (see Chapter 4). An extensive series of longitudinal studies by Allaman, Joyce, and Crandall (1972) investigated developmental antecedents of individual differences in need for approval (often called approval motivation). Their work identified a rather clear-cut set of predictors of need for approval which centered around the practices that parents use in raising their children. In general, children who scored high on the Children's Social Desirability Scale (a measure of approval motivation for children) tended to have parents who employed relatively harsh modes of child rearing. Specifically, mothers of high need for approval children tended to be less warm and affectionate, praised their children less, punished them more, and were more restrictive. The relationship between these parental behaviors and children's need for approval was quite strong; maternal behavior predicted 60-80% of the variance in need for approval scores in one study. In addition, perceived rejection by the father was correlated with high need for approval in young men.

Allaman et al. conclude that parenting practices that communicate disinterest, disapproval, or rejection to the child create a generalized concern with others' evaluations and a strong desire for approval and acceptance from their parents and others. Much of the behavior of high need for approval individuals can be interpreted as attempts to obtain approval and avoid disapproval (see Strickland, 1977, for a review). Unfortunately, children of disapproving, rejecting parents not only are highly motivated to gain approval, but they are also likely to develop a generalized low expectancy of actually obtaining it. Allaman et al. (1972, p. 1156) foreshadow the self-presentation approach to social anxiousness by noting that "a combination of high value for approval (or avoidance of disapproval), but a low expectancy of obtaining it results in apprehension in evaluative situations."

SELF-ESTEEM

Self-esteem correlates more highly with social anxiousness than any other construct that has been examined (e.g., Cheek & Buss, 1981; Clark & Arkowitz, 1975; Leary, 1983a; McCroskey, 1977; Zimbardo, 1977). People who are low in self-esteem are much more likely to experience social anxiety than those with higher self-esteem.

Most psychologists consider it axiomatic that a primary determinant of the self-concept and self-esteem is found in reflected appraisals. Reflected appraisals are a person's beliefs regarding how he or she is perceived and evaluated by other people. Others' perceived reactions are a primary source of information about oneself. Am I a good swimmer? Am I smart? Am I pretty? Do I sing well? Such questions are answered, in part, by the evaluatively tainted responses of others toward the individual. Others' appraisals are a particularly important source of self-information when objective criteria for self-evaluation are not available (Festinger, 1954).

The effect of reflected appraisals on self-esteem are particularly dramatic in childhood. New self-images are developing at a rapid rate and the child has few internalized standards or objective criteria for self-evaluation. Inasmuch as this is true, it is not surprising that parents have a strong impact upon their children's self-concepts and self-esteem. Consciously and unconsciously, parents convey their impressions and evaluations of the child—judgments that may subsequently be internalized by the child. Thus, people who think they are accepted and liked by their parents tend to accept and like themselves (Helper, 1955; Jourard & Remy, 1955). It follows, then, that child-rearing styles that convey parental acceptance of the child should tend to produce children with higher self-esteem than those that convey nonacceptance.

It is difficult to fit parenting styles into neat categories, but for our purposes it will be convenient to refer to a classical scheme proposed by Baumrind (1971). Baumrind classifies child-rearing styles into three types. *Permissive* parents are relatively nondemanding of their children, providing the child with as much freedom and autonomy as possible. The child is given a great deal of choice in most matters, rules are few and enforced inconsistently, and permissive parents seldom provide guidelines for their children to follow. In contrast, *authoritarian* parents are highly controlling, directive, and restrictive. They have many strict rules that are enforced stringently. Deviations from carefully prescribed behavior are not tolerated, and children have little, if any, input into decisions that affect them. In addition, authoritarian parents tend to favor punishment-based rather than reinforcement-based discipline. *Authoritative* parents evidence a combination of the permissive and authoritarian styles. Although they have high standards for their children and enforce them consistently, authoritative parents tend to allow their children as much freedom as the child is able to handle at any given age. The child's opinions are valued, particularly regarding decisions that affect the child. Discipline is typically reward-oriented and rational, designed to help the child understand the reasons for appropriate behavior. Authoritative parents insist upon children behaving properly, but punish rule-infractions less severely than either permissive or authoritarian parents.

In general, parents who use an authoritative approach to raising their children are more likely to have children with relatively high self-esteem who are less prone to feelings of social anxiety (Coopersmith, 1967; Zimbardo, 1981). To understand why, let us examine a few specific differences among the three parenting styles with an eye toward the possible effects of these differences on the child's self-esteem and social confidence.

Coopersmith (1967) conducted what is probably the most extensive investigation of the antecedents of self-esteem in children. Not surprisingly, he found that parents of high self-esteem children tend to be more warmly accepting of their children than parents of low self-esteem children. Parents of high self-esteemers are more concerned with their children's lives and problems, interested in and encouraging of their children's pursuits, know and like their children's friends better, and enjoy their offspring more. They are also more affectionate toward their children and more accessible when their children need them. A moment's thought will show that this orientation, adopted most often by authoritative parents, conveys to the child that their parents consider them significant, valuable, and loveable individuals, worthy of others' attention, esteem, and acceptance. Children of cold, aloof, disinterested, and/or rejecting parents are likely to conclude that they are undesirable individuals, unworthy of others' care and concern. Permissive parents are likely to foster this impression through apparent lack of concern. Authoritarian parents may appear rejecting and disapproving because of their strictness and punitiveness.

The three styles of parenting differ also in the degree to which they balance the child's autonomy against a parent-provided structure. By giving the child as much freedom and responsibility as possible, authoritative parents foster a sense of self-sufficiency in their children. The children of authoritative parents learn they can take care of themselves. Permissive and authoritarian parents, on the other hand, stunt their chldren's sense of control and self-sufficiency. The permissive parent does not provide enough guidance and structure to assure that the child learns appropriate and functional ways of dealing with life. Authoritarian parents prevent their children from gaining the experience needed to build self-confidence by dictating most of their children's actions. In short, the authoritative approach avoids both the implicit lack of concern of permissive parents and the controlling punitiveness of authoritarian parents—both of which diminish self-esteem and self-confidence (Coopersmith, 1967; Rosenberg, 1965).

High self-esteem people also tend to have parents who clearly accept their independence, individualism, and opinions (Coopersmith, 1967). Their parents are willing to consider the child's voice in family decisions, tolerate reasonable objections from the child, compromise with the child when appropriate, and use rational discussions rather than force to enforce decisions. This is contrasted with the permissive parent who always allows the child freedom regardless of the consequences, and authoritarian parents who do not consider the child's perspective at all, tolerate no objections to parental authority, and use punishment to enforce their mandates. By conveying to the child that his or her voice is important, the authoritative parent projects respect and confidence for the child that heightens self-esteem.

Of course, parents are not the only shapers of their children's identities and self-esteem. School teachers and personnel also play a major role (Kash & Borich, 1978). There is a correlation between children's perceptions of their teacher's feelings toward them and their perceptions of themselves (Davidson & Lang, 1960). We have all squirmed in our seats when, as students, the teacher berated another child in front of the class: "What's wrong, Billy? Do I have to draw a picture for you? Maybe we should send you back to kindergarten until you're ready for fifth grade." Few teachers intend to be cruel, but the frustration of the job leads even the best to belittle students as a way of enforcing compliance, shaming students into working harder, or controlling the classroom. The toll of such behaviors on student self-esteem is immense. Davidson and Lang (1960) argue that "it is essential that teachers communicate positive feelings to their children and thus not only strengthen their self appraisals but stimulate their growth academically as well as interpersonally." As with parents, teachers may foster high self-esteem via respect for and acceptance of the student as an individual, the setting of reasonable limits, consistent enforcement of necessary rules, and inviting students' input into decisions that affect them.

Most studies of self-esteem have focused on people's overall self-evaluations. Of course, people may evaluate different aspects of themselves in different ways. Even a high self-esteem individual may evaluate one or more *specific* aspects of him- or herself unfavorably. If these specific attributes are perceived as central to making particular, desired impressions on others, even an otherwise high self-esteem individual may experience social anxiety.

These brief observations demonstrate the kinds of social and psychological factors that influence individual differences in self-esteem and thereby affect individual differences in social anxiousness. Future research should focus more directly on the relationship between parenting styles and social anxiety.

SOCIAL SKILLS

Social skills are learned. No one is born prepared to perform the wide variety of behaviors that are needed to navigate the sometimes treacherous waters of social life. Socially skilled responses are learned and refined throughout life although the rudiments of such behaviors are probably acquired in childhood and adolescence. People who for one reason or another do not learn socially facilitative ways of interacting are at a disadvantage in social encounters and may come to perceive that they are not as socially skilled as other people they know. This realization may lead individuals to doubt that they can perform competently in certain kinds of encounters or make favorable impressions on others when socially skilled behaviors are called for. As we saw earlier, a great deal of research shows that self-perceived skill deficits may precipitate social anxiety.

How are social behaviors learned? As with most complex actions, social responses are acquired through observation and modeling (Bandura, 1973). For children, the most potent models for many behaviors are parents. As a result, parents who are not particularly socially adroit will not provide appropriate models for their children to emulate. Not only will children of socially unskilled parents fail to observe frequent instances of skilled behaviors, but they may actually imitate examples of inappropriate, nonfacilitative social responses. When a child sees a parent falter nervously in social situations, use annoying or ambiguous nonverbal gestures, speak too fast or too slowly for maximal communication, or fail to provide the social cues that facilitate contingent interactions, the child will not learn the most skillful ways of responding and, possibly, will mimic the parent's unskilled behavior. Children of socially competent, confident, and poised parents, however, have models from which to learn more adaptive social responses.

Filsinger and Lamke (1983) have conducted one of the few studies investigating the link between social difficulties in parents and their children. In their study, college students and their parents completed the Social Avoidance and Distress (SAD) Scale and the Dyadic Adjustment Scale (a measure of interpersonal competence in intimate relationships). Mothers' SAD scores correlated positively with their children's SAD scores and negatively with their children's interpersonal competence, suggesting that socially anxious and avoidant mothers tend to raise children who also have social difficulties. There were no correlations between fathers' and children's scores on the two measures. Clearly, a great deal more research on parents' effects on children's social anxiety and skill is needed.

In addition to modeling social behavior, some parents directly instruct their children regarding important social skills. Children may be taught to converse more effectively, the appropriate uses of nonverbal gestures, the skill of being a good listener, politeness, and so on.

Like all learned behaviors, social behaviors require practice to make perfect. Parents who frequently talk with (not *to*) their children and who encourage their children to express themselves openly and honestly provide them with needed practice. Similarly,

Wicklund, R. A. Objective self-awareness. In L. Berkowitz (Ed.), *Advances in experimental social psychology* (Vol. 8). New York: Academic Press, 1975.

Wilkins, W. Desensitization: Social and cognitive factors underlying the effectiveness of Wolpe's procedure. *Psychological Bulletin,* 1971, *76,* 311-317.

Wine, J. D. Test anxiety and direction of attention. *Psychological Bulletin,* 1971, *76,* 92-104.

Wolpe, J. *Psychotherapy by reciprocal inhibition.* Stanford: Stanford University Press, 1958.

Wolpe. J. *The practice of behavior therapy.* New York: Pergammon, 1973.

Wrightsman, L. S. Effects of waiting with others on changes in felt level of anxiety. *Journal of Abnormal and Social Psychology,* 1960, *61,* 216-222.

Zaidel, S., & Mehrabian, A. The ability to communicate and infer positive and negative attitudes facially and verbally. *Journal of Experimental Research in Personality,* 1969, *3,* 233-241.

Zimbardo, P. G. *Shyness: What it is and what to do about it.* New York: Jove, 1977.

Zimbardo, P. G. *Cognitive and cultural contributions to shyness and loneliness.* Paper presented at the meeting of the American Psychological Association, Montreal, 1980.

Zimbardo, P. G. *The shy child.* New York: McGraw-Hill, 1981.

Zimbardo, P. G., Pilkonis, P. A., & Norwood, R. M. *The silent prison of shyness.* Office of Naval Research Tech. Report Z-17, Stanford University, 1974.

NAME INDEX

SUBJECT INDEX

ABOUT THE AUTHOR

MARK R. LEARY, Ph.D., is Assistant Professor in the Department of Educational Psychology at the University of Texas at Austin. He received his doctorate in social psychology from the University of Florida in 1980 and taught for three years at Denison University. In addition to the study of social anxiety, his current interests include self-presentation, social cognition, and integrations of social and clinical-counseling psychology.